# massage
## TO GO

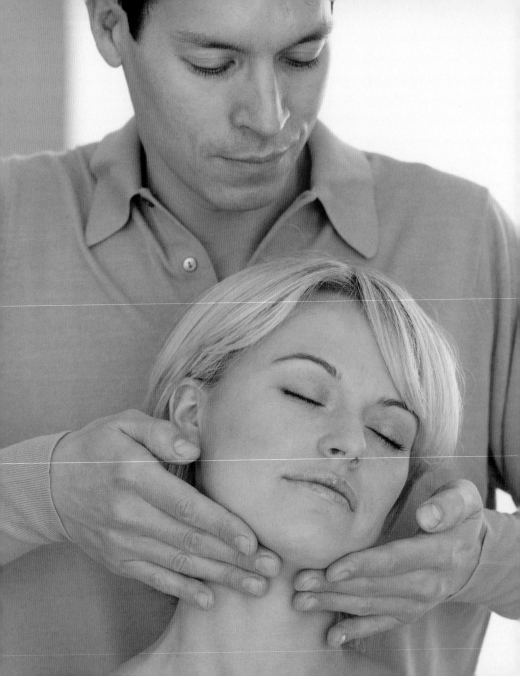

# massage
## TO GO

**Eileen Bentley**

An Hachette Livre UK Company

First published in Great Britain in 2008 by
Gaia Books, a division of Octopus Publishing Group Ltd
2–4 Heron Quays, London E14 4JP
www.octopusbooks.co.uk

This material was previously published as *A Gaia Busy Person's Guide: Massage*

ISBN: 978-1-85675-297-8

A CIP catalogue record for this book is available from the British Library

Printed and bound in China

10 9 8 7 6 5 4 3 2 1

**Cautionary note:**
All reasonable care has been taken in the preparation of this book, but the information it contains is not meant to take the place of medical care under the direct supervision of a doctor. Before making any changes in your health regime, always consult a doctor. While all the therapies detailed in this book are completely safe if done correctly, you must seek professional advice if you are in any doubt about any medical condition.  Any application of the ideas and information contained in this book is at the reader's sole discretion and risk.

**Direction** Lyn Hemming, Patrick Nugent
**Production** Jim Pope, Louise Hall
**Editors** Fiona Biggs, Kelly Thomson
**Design** Phil Gamble
**Photography** Ruth Jenkinson

# Contents

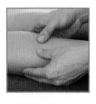 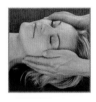 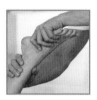 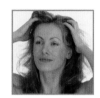

Using this book                                          6
Introduction                                             8

**CHAPTER ONE: GETTING STARTED**                        10

**CHAPTER TWO: PREPARATION FOR THE DAY**                28

**CHAPTER THREE: MASSAGE ON THE MOVE**                  48

**CHAPTER FOUR: MASSAGE AT WORK**                       60

**CHAPTER FIVE: RELAXING WITH HEAD MASSAGE**            78

**CHAPTER SIX: THE WHOLE WORKS**                        92

Further reading                                        123
Index                                                  124
Acknowledgements                                       127

# Using this book

This book offers a selection of massage techniques drawn from Shiatsu, head massage, acupressure, aromatherapy, therapeutic massage, meditation, and the use of crystals in re-balancing energy, to take you through busy days and into relaxing evenings. You can use it to guide you into a daily calming routine that will help to energize and revitalize your life, or you can dip into it to discover quick ways to defuse a tense situation, to overcome afternoon tiredness, or to help alleviate the daily aches and pains that can adversely affect your performance.

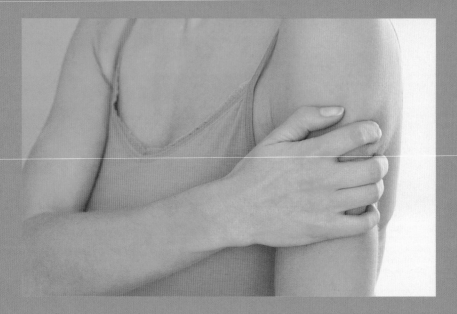

Basic techniques are explained in Chapter One. You will learn how to use your hands, your arms, and even your feet to bring good health and well-being to you and your partner. You are also introduced to different therapies and exercises and the role of crystals in helping to maintain a good balance of energy.

Chapter Two takes you through a daily routine that will help to get you started for the busy day. This covers breathing and exercises to wake up every cell in your body. It also includes self-help routines for some of the more common ailments that can strike because of stress, the daily use of computers, difficulties at work, and the build-up of tensions during the average day. It ends with a chakra meditation, which, if practised regularly, will transform your life by re-charging your body's energy centres, removing any sense of lack in your life, improving your creativity and awareness, and calming your mind and body.

Chapters Three and Four deal with your daily working life, from travelling to work, through various times where you can take short re-energizing massage breaks, to the later part of the day when you may need some real help with headache, tiredness, and lack of concentration.

Chapter Five takes you into the evening at home, where you and your partner can start the process of relaxation by giving each other a head massage.

Chapter Six provides the techniques for a long, relaxing full body massage session that will totally de-stress and relax you both, ready for the next day.

**THE POWER OF TOUCH**
*Good diet, regular exercise, and massage are well-established ways of boosting the body's own healing powers, energy, and resistance to disease. Even if you do become ill, regular massage will speed recovery.*

# Introduction

The healing, communicative, and bonding power of touch has been very well understood down through the centuries. All cultures, civilizations, and communities, human or animal, have used touch as a means of communication and bringing their society together.

Touch is not only a comforting and pleasurable means of relaxing; it is also a very necessary part of being alive. Research with institutionalized orphans has shown that denying touch is very detrimental to the basic health of the child. Those who were touched, even if they had succumbed to serious illness, were brought back to and maintained good health. Other studies included those undergoing major surgery and suffering life-threatening and long-term illness. In each case, including massage in their treatment resulted in faster, less painful, and longer-lasting recovery.

## WHAT IS MASSAGE?

From the desire to touch and be touched sprang many, varied therapies. Some use only the simplest touch of holding a hand and wishing, or channelling, good health and well-being to the one being treated.

Others are elaborate, energetic, even gymnastic in their approach. However, as the great Shiatsu master Shizuto Masunaga has said, "When you begin, you give long technical treatments. When you get better, your treatments get shorter." So, a few well-spent moments of treatment done with care and good intention can bring just as many benefits as a long routine executed with precision.

So what exactly is massage? It has been described as the restoration and maintenance of good health by means of manipulation of the body's soft tissue. That's the short answer. Massage is also a holistic therapy, which considers the whole person, their choices of food, drink, occupation, and pastimes. With a wide variety of disciplines from which to choose, there is treatment or therapy to suit every person or problem.

## HOW IT WORKS

Some massage therapies work on muscles, joints, ligaments, and tendons. They work firmly to move tissue over tissue, so ridding the body of the toxic build-up that can cause physical problems such as arthritis, rheumatism, and sciatica. Others work in a more gentle way, reaching far within the body's energy systems to release deep-rooted problems. Even entrenched emotional problems can be moved and cleared out of your body and mind by sensitive massage.

Is it dangerous? Messing about with your mind as well as your body may sound frightening. Many people will run from exposing their innermost feelings. Even though you may sometimes feel a little emotionally wobbly after a massage you will always be in control of yourself. This is a normal reaction and it will clear up after a few days. You may even find that deep-rooted problems will surface and clear and this will cause you to feel much more alive and free.

## LEARNING THE TECHNIQUES

To enable you to treat specific ailments or problems you should undertake a professional training course in whichever therapy you choose to study. However, to give a massage that will very effectively release everyday problems that have no medical cause, you don't need any professional training. Working gently, with loving care, while wishing good health and well-being to yourself or the person you are working on will prepare you to meet life's next challenge.

## TAKING CARE OF YOURSELF

If you are going to look after the health and well-being of others you must first look after yourself. It is very important to constantly refresh your own levels of energy to avoid becoming worn-out, depleted, or ill. Regular practice of breathing, meditation, and bodywork such as arm swinging will help you to develop your basic fitness, awareness, ability to focus and concentrate, stamina, flexibility, and reflexes. Even if you are only working on yourself, regular practice of the exercises will improve your techniques and deepen the effectiveness of the massage.

Eilean Bentley

# CHAPTER ONE

# Getting started

Massage needs no special equipment. You don't even need to use your hands. Many therapists use only their feet and knees. And you don't need to take your clothes off. In fact, for many massage therapies it is better to wear light clothing to provide a barrier between the giver and the receiver, since the touch of bare skin can distract the giver from a full awareness of the body's energy.

Regular massage can relieve stress, tension, tiredness, aching joints, headaches, insomnia, digestive problems, and emotionally related disturbances such as Crohn's disease, irritable bowel syndrome (IBS), and asthma. Massage is relaxing, pleasurable, bonding, and regenerating. It can help you to clear your thoughts, increase your creativity, open your awareness, lose weight, release depression, strengthen joints, loosen muscles, stretch tendons, increase overall flexibility, and much more. The healing power of massage is greatly enhanced by combining it with meditation and visualization, encouraging the receiver's own healing intentions to support the giver. Using essential oils and crystals can increase the potency of the treatment.

When you arrive at work, mentally build into your day at least one 30-minute break where you can give yourself a revitalizing workout with head massage, loosening exercises, and calming breathing exercises.

If you find yourself daydreaming it means that you need a break to gather your thoughts. Turn your daydreams into short meditations and take a few moments to massage your neck or shoulders. Try to get away from your phones and computer for 15 minutes to recharge your batteries. Take another quick refresher at the close of the day, before you set off for home. It will calm you before you have to tackle rush-hour chaos. Have a good, relaxing massage at least twice a week to regenerate your whole being.

# Techniques

Here are a few basic techniques to get you started. Once you have mastered the general principles you may find that you start making up your own strokes and sequences. Go with what feels good for you and your partner. Don't worry too much about the right way or the wrong way, just go.

■ *Stroking* Use flat hands, fingers, thumbs, even your forearms, in a smooth, flowing action, running lightly over the body in straight lines, circles, or long sweeps. You can use both hands together, covering a large area such as the back, or one hand after the other, giving a continuous flow of following strokes. Place your hands (or fingers, thumbs, or forearms) on the area being worked and glide lightly over the surface, in your chosen direction.

■ *Rotations* Using firm pressure, work your fingers, thumbs, or elbows in small circles over one spot.

■ *Kneading* Good for large muscles over the shoulders and back, but can be used in other areas if you moderate the pressure. Use your fist or the heel of your hand against the pressure of your other palm, thumbs working against fingers, or fingers against thumbs, in a pinching action that works a large area.

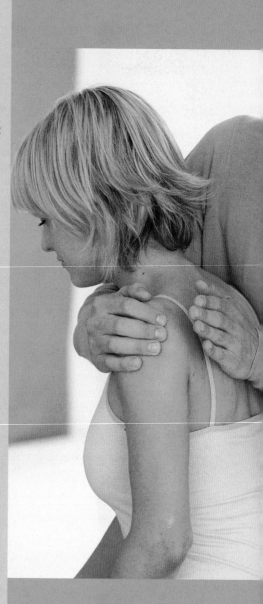

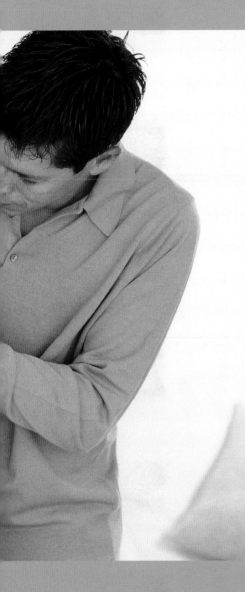

The pressure should be firm but never to the point of pain.

■ *Pinching* Similar to kneading, but you pick up small areas of flesh between your fingers and thumbs. Again, be firm without causing any actual pain.

■ *Wringing* Taking the muscle between both hands, twist your hands in opposite directions. This is just like wringing out wet towels. It should work the muscle fibres together without pain.

■ *Pressure* Use your fingers, thumbs, fists, elbows, feet, knees, or any part of your body that can exert a still, steady pressure on the relevant area to master this energy-toning technique.

■ *Hacking/tapping/pummelling* You can use the sides of your hands or the backs of your hands (hacking), your fingertips (tapping), your fist, or clasped hands (pummelling). This is a rapid drumming movement, using one hand after the other, or, in the case of your clasped hands, both hands together. The pressure varies from light tapping to heavy pummelling, with hacking coming somewhere in between.

■ *Knuckling* Usually you use the large knuckles of your fingers, but you can also use the smaller knuckles to work more delicate areas, such as the face.

# Different types of massage

The techniques in this book have been drawn from a variety of massages. This is not a comprehensive study of each massage, more a selection of moves, pressure points, and steps, which can be quickly and easily used by any beginner.

### SHIATSU (01)
This is a slow, gentle, relaxing form of massage. All that may seem to be going on is someone leaning with their fingers, thumbs, or arms on another person or gently wringing their limbs. However, the power of Shiatsu is deep. Positive intention is all-important – this is how the practitioner controls the direction and strength of the energy passing through the recipient. Working on tsubos (vital Japanese pressure points) while focusing on the inner energy channels (meridians) of the receiver, the giver slowly releases unhealthy blockages and rebalances the flow of energy within the body.

### HEAD MASSAGE (02)
Massaging your head, neck, and shoulders releases tension in the muscles of the upper body, relieving headaches, destressing your mind and body, and moving toxins out of your system. Working the tsubos on the many meridians within this area can improve the health of the internal organs, and tone and refresh your whole being.

### AROMATHERAPY
For many centuries healers have used the essences of plants to assist in the curing of many ailments. Aromatherapy is a very relaxing, pleasurable way of absorbing those powerful, healing oils into our bodies. There is an oil for almost every problem, and combining oils with the power of touch results in a therapy that is one of the most relaxing, calming, and refreshing ways to unwind after a busy day.

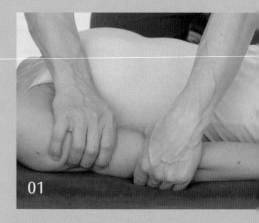

01

## ACUPRESSURE (03)

Unlike Shiatsu, which works on meridians and pressure points that are not necessarily in fixed positions, acupressure and acupuncture both use fixed points. They can be activated by a firm touch, a needle (in the case of acupuncture), or an electrical current. The pressure points are very responsive and can relieve pain, sickness, and stiffness in muscles and joints very quickly and effectively. To get the best from an acupressure treatment you must apply firm pressure for at least a minute to each point used.

## THERAPEUTIC MASSAGE

For deep muscle, joint, and other problems, the strong manipulative techniques of therapeutic massage can bring great relief. The intention of the giver is fixed on the structure of your body, so that they are aware of underlying problems within muscles, organs, and the skeletal, digestive, circulatory, and nervous systems. The healing work relies on the movement of tissue over tissue, which releases toxic waste build-up from your muscles and joints. Therapeutic massage, with its medical origins, is more clinical than the more ancient and traditional systems of Shiatsu and acupressure.

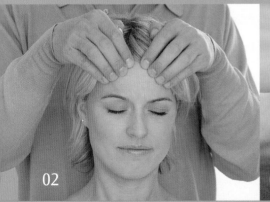

02

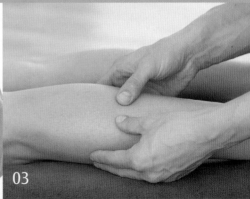

03

# Pressure points for massage

Acupressure points are not magic buttons that can turn health problems off like a light switch. But used regularly and with care, they can rebalance the health of your body and mind so that the problems become less frequent in occurrence and intensity.

Having said that, sometimes the points can work swiftly and effectively to ease a problem. I have treated people with back pain, headaches, tension-related sickness, and breathing and mobility problems, whose symptoms have apparently cleared up immediately. However, in many cases, it has been a first aid treatment – it alleviated symptoms, but didn't deal with the underlying problem, which required care and further treatment.

The danger with "push-button" cures is that you will overstrain your system by returning too quickly to your old ways, and the problem that prompted you to seek treatment will return. Pain and sickness are often lifestyle problems. The acupressure points here can help only as an addition to good posture, healthy eating, good sleep, relaxed mind, and positive mental habits and practices.

**FOR THE TOP OF THE HEAD AND THE BACK OF THE BODY**

■ *GV20* Poor memory and concentration, headaches, mild depression. Clears the brain and calms the mind.

■ *GV16* Colds, headaches, sore throats, nosebleeds.

■ *GB20* Stiff neck, tension headaches, insomnia, hypertension. Use with GV16 to help relieve the symptoms of colds.

■ *B10* Stress, tension, anxiety, insomnia. Opens the awareness, calms the mind, relaxes the body, relieves colds and flu.

■ *GB21* Tension and tiredness in the shoulders and neck, frozen shoulder. Relaxes the mind, reduces nervous stress, anger, irritability. Very energizing.

■ *B13* Breathing difficulties, detoxifying.

■ *B23, B47* Relieve lower backache, rebalance energy in the kidneys and digestive system.

■ *TH4* Soothes wrist pain.

■ *LI4* Headaches, mild depression, general pain. Anaesthetic and detoxifying.

■ *K3* Water retention, swollen feet, sleeping difficulties. Protects the immune system. Very useful and safe in pregnancy, eases labour.

■ *B60* Lower back pain, joint and rheumatic pain in the lower body.

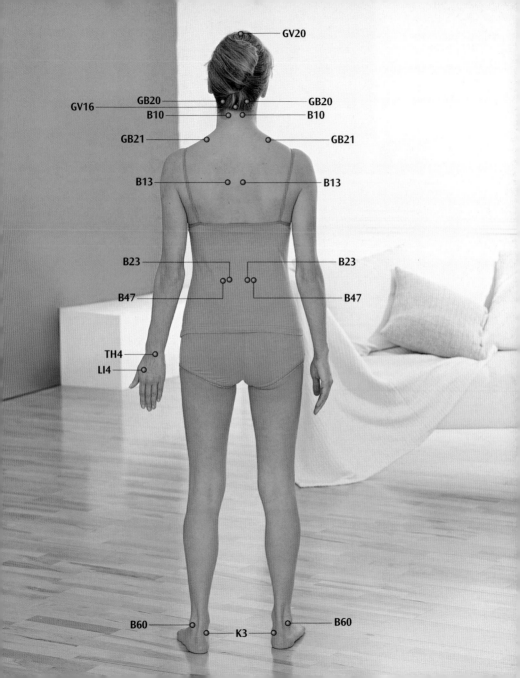

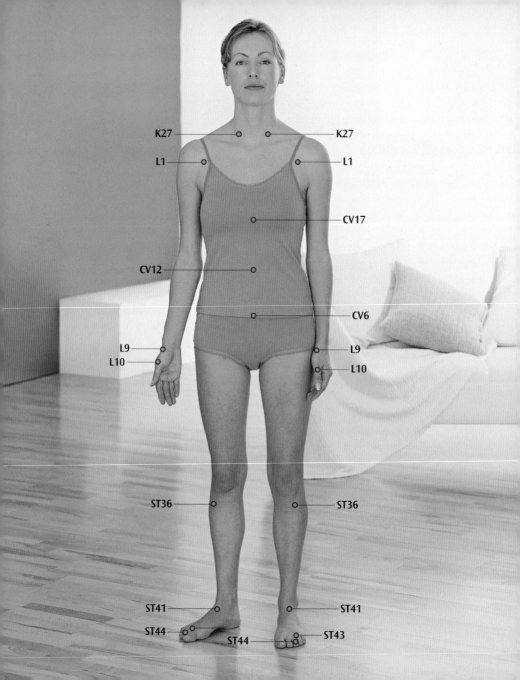

K27 —————○ ○————— K27

L1 —————○ ○————— L1

CV17 ———○

CV12 ———○

CV6 ———○

L9 ——○ ○—— L9
L10 —○ ○— L10

ST36 —○ ○— ST36

ST41 —○ ○— ST41
ST44 —○
ST44 ——— ○— ST43

## FOR THE FACE AND THE FRONT OF THE BODY

- *GV25* Depression, weak immune system. Clears the mind, calms fears, relaxes the body.
- *B2, GV24.5* Eye and sinus problems, headaches, and other facial pain.
- *B1* Nosebleeds, tired and aching eyes.
- *LI20* Head colds, nasal congestion.
- *ST2* Good for the complexion, relieves eye strain.
- *ST3* Sinuses, tired, dry eyes.
- *GV26* Dizziness, fainting, cramp.
- *K27* Sore throat, coughing, hiccups, anxiety. Rebalances the kidneys.
- *L1* Asthma, breathing difficulties. Stabilizes the emotions, eases confusion, clears the mind.

- *CV17* Mild depression, grief.
- *CV12* Emotional problems, stress, digestive problems.
- *CV6* Trapped wind, constipation, lower back problems. Revitalizes the body's energy flow.
- *L9* Relieves asthma, bronchitis. Reduces fear, anger, anxiety.
- *L10* Lung congestion, emotional upset, wrist pain.
- *ST36* Sickness, nausea. Balances the digestive system, stimulates the immune system, boosts energy.
- *ST41* Fear, nervous tension. Ankle and heel pain.
- *ST43, ST44* Excess wind, sickness and nausea, facial pain, nosebleeds, aching teeth and gums.

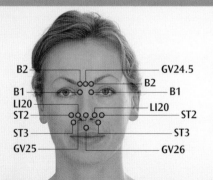

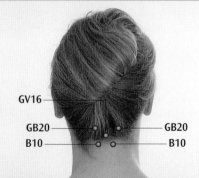

# Aromatherapy massage

An aromatherapy massage, either as a self-treatment or working with a partner, is a simple, extremely effective way to unwind at the end of a day. The techniques are very safe and easy to use. They are mainly long, smooth, stroking movements, done with the flat palms, fingers, thumbs, and sometimes the forearms, working on bare skin. This technique combines the senses of touch and smell to give a relaxing, calming treatment.

You don't need a special working surface such as a couch – you can work on the floor on folded blankets covered by a sheet. This allows you to use your body weight to increase the strength of the stroke but still gives the feeling of rhythmic effortlessness.

**CAUTION**
- *Do not use oil on the eyes as this may irritate the delicate tissues.*
- *Do not exert strong pressure on the soft tissue of the abdomen.*

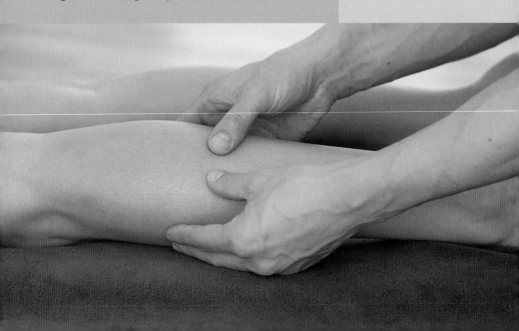

## OILS

Always dilute essential oils in a carrier oil (grapeseed, sunflower, sweet almond, sesame, soya) for massage. The usual proportions are 15 drops of essential oil to 60ml of carrier oil for a full-body massage. For a smaller area such as the face use 5 drops to 30ml.

- *Angelica* Calming, good for digestion, antiseptic, antiviral. Do not use during pregnancy. Photo-toxic, so avoid exposure to sunlight after use.
- *Chamomile* Relaxing, anti-inflammatory.
- *Citronella* Good for aches and pains. Also good as an insect repellent. Do not use this oil during pregnancy.
- *Clary sage* Warming and soothing. Do not use this oil during pregnancy.
- *Eucalyptus* Antiseptic, decongestant, antiviral.
- *Frankincense* Warming, relaxing, uplifting.
- *Geranium* Soothing, relaxing, antidepressant.
- *Jasmine* Uplifting, relaxing, good for cramp.
- *Lavender* Soothing, relaxing, antiseptic.
- *Lemon* Refreshing, stimulating, antiseptic. Photo-toxic, so avoid exposure to sunlight after use.
- *Myrrh* Warming, relaxing, anti-inflammatory. Do not use this oil during pregnancy.
- *Peppermint* Cooling, good for digestion, mentally stimulating. Never use undiluted or before sleeping.
- *Petitgrain* Soothing, calming, antidepressant.
- *Rosemary* Stimulating, refreshing. Do not use this oil during pregnancy or if you suffer from epilepsy.
- *Tea tree* Antifungal, antiseptic.
- *Ylang-ylang* Euphoric, aphrodisiac, relaxing. Use in moderation.

# Aromatherapy: basic strokes

## STROKING (01)

You can use strong pressure on the back of the body –
for the legs use your palms, fingers, and fists; for the
back you can also use your forearms. You can use both
hands together or one hand after the other, keeping
up a continuous rhythm. Work from feet to knees,
repeating the stroke three or four times. Then work
from knees to buttocks in the same way, then up over
the back and up the backs of the arms. You can also
work in the opposite direction, starting at the
shoulders, moving down the arms, the back, and,
finally, the legs. Work systematically and rhythmically.

When stroking the front of the body, start at the
shoulders and work down the arms, then down the
front of the chest to the abdomen. You can use a
stronger pressure over the front of the legs, down to
the feet. Use a firm stroke on the feet as a light touch
can tickle and this is not relaxing.

When massaging yourself or a partner, use only
your fingers on the face, moving in a light upward
direction. Starting under the chin, stroke up to the
temples three or four times, then across the lips and
under the nose, across the nose to the temple area,
and across the forehead from the centre to the sides.

## RAKING

Using the pads of your fingertips rake upward over the
legs and arms. Rake over the back from side to spine,
one side at a time. Use firm but not hard pressure,
and the lightest pressure over the face.

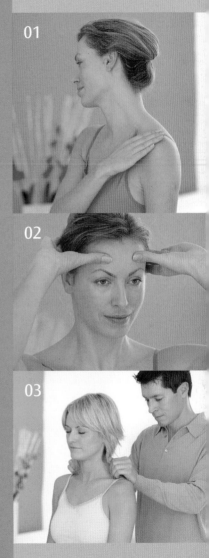

## THUMB ROTATIONS AND PRESSURE (02)

For rotations, move your thumb(s) in small circles to work firmly into the area. For pressure, drop your weight on to your thumbs and hold for a few moments. With a lighter hold, you can also use rotations and pressure over the neck and facial area.

## KNEADING (03)

For strongly muscled areas, support your partner's body with one hand and, using firm pressure with the fist of your other hand, slide your fist over the body toward your supporting hand. On all other areas use your thumbs, sliding in a firm pressure toward your outstretched fingers in a pinching action.

## FRICTION RUB

Rub the palms or edges of your hands over your partner's body with an alternate sawing action, one hand after the other.

## PUMMELLING/HACKING

The strongest action is with two hands clasped together and used to pound the flesh. Using your hands individually, one after the other, will give a rapid drumming treatment. Cupped hands or fingers are the lightest and are most suitable for more sensitive areas.

# Crystals and massage

Many therapists are achieving very good results by giving their clients crystals to hold during treatment. The crystals seem to deepen the treatment and relax and clear not only the person being treated, but also the person giving the treatment. After all, our bodies and minds are crystals in solution. Even the solid matter of tissue forms crystals if it is dried, and our spirit is pure energy.

Crystals are also very beneficial for the energy of the room in which they are placed. All stones work at their best when they are in the environment in which they were formed. Their energies are complemented fully by all that is around them. They are at home. However, it is not usually practical for many people to go to the home of a crystal. The crystals must travel to you. During that journey they can pick up many energies, from the person who mined or found them, right through the many transactions that eventually brought them to you. Neutralizing these energies is a necessary process through which they must go if you are to be able to access their properties free from any other influence.

There are many ways of doing this. You can run them under cold water to earth the energy. If you have a collection of crystals you can cleanse any new ones by surrounding them with your existing collection. You can also cleanse them by placing your energy within them. Hold the stone in your hand and visualize your hands filling with light. See the crystal absorbing the light and releasing any negativity. Earth this negativity by visualizing it flowing down into the ground. This is a good method to use if you are going to programme the stones for a specific purpose, such as healing. The way I prefer is to wrap the stones in a natural material, such as cotton, and bury them in the garden for a few days. This has the advantage of balancing their energies with those of the land about them. It gives them a new home.

The relationship between a crystal and its holder is very like the relationship between two people. It depends upon the qualities of both to make a whole, and these qualities can be different in different relationships. So a stone that works in one way for your friend may not work in quite the same way with you, or even in the same way as it did with you under different circumstances. To find which stone is right for you at any one time, you must spend a few moments connecting with the stones. Hold them, one at a time, in your hand and see how you feel. Try out a selection, and work with the one that feels most in tune with the way you need to progress. For example, if you feel tired and depressed then an old favourite, amethyst, may not be right for you this time, as it is a transforming stone and could be too changeable for your mood. Try rose quartz first to calm and clear your emotions or malachite to clear your mind and raise your energy levels. However, amethyst could be the right stone if you need to make decisions that could bring change into your life.

A word of caution – if you have any mental health problems crystals can trigger unwanted reactions.

# A selection of crystals

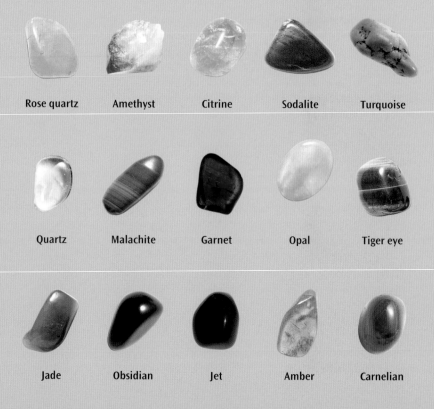

Rose quartz    Amethyst    Citrine    Sodalite    Turquoise

Quartz    Malachite    Garnet    Opal    Tiger eye

Jade    Obsidian    Jet    Amber    Carnelian

Here are a few crystals you might like to try. These descriptions are not comprehensive, merely a guide.

- *Rose quartz* Calming, cooling influence, releases negativity.
- *Amethyst* Balances the mental, emotional, and physical bodies, good for life-changing decisions.
- *Citrine* Balancing, used for aligning the chakras and harmonizing the yin and yang energies.
- *Sodalite* Aids logical thought, releases confusion, good for group work.
- *Turquoise* Strengthens and harmonizes the chakras, facilitates communication and intuition.
- *Quartz* Used for healing, protection, space-clearing. Dispels static electricity. Brings clarity of mind.
- *Malachite* Clears the mind, aids logical thought processes.
- *Garnet* Increases steadiness of thought and action, dependability, and orderliness.
- *Opal* Intensifies powers of perception, awakens creativity. Best used with a protective stone such as carnelian to temper its excesses.

- *Tiger eye* Opens you to awareness of your true needs and the needs of others. Releases relationship fears, encourages openness toward others.
- *Jade* Brings gentle peace and harmony to mind and spirit. Enhances intuition. Encourages psychic awareness and receptivity.
- *Obsidian* Helps to develop inner vision and clarity. Protective. Helps you to find strength in adversity.
- *Jet* Very protective, calms the mind, dispels unnecessary fears, reduces depression, enhances stability.
- *Amber* Clears energy, lightens moods, opens you to unconditional love.
- *Carnelian* Neutralizes negative feelings, encourages loving feelings toward all. Very useful if you wish to move on to working with more dynamic stones as it protects you from the initial rush of enthusiasms and excesses often generated by them.

# CHAPTER TWO

# Preparation for the day

Plan to get up half an hour or so earlier than you usually do. Waking up slowly, instead of leaping out of bed at the last minute will give your body and mind the opportunity to synchronize. Your muscles will have time to warm up and your mind will clear in readiness for whatever the day brings.

Begin your day before you get out of bed with some stretches and energy-clearing stroking. Then indulge in some energizing massage in your shower. Combine this with a mind- and body-clearing meditation and you will be powered up even before you've had breakfast.

Play games while you are dressing. Feel the action of every muscle, every fibre, every cell. Make it a dance. Be aware of all that you can see, feel the colours. Try to hear every birdsong, the fridge starting up, passing cars. Pretend you are writing a TV script. Describe to yourself everything around you. If you do this often enough you will become bored with the same descriptions and you'll start to find greater depths in everything. This simple exercise will develop your powers of observation and speed up your ability to think in multiple ways.

Appreciate every mouthful of your breakfast. This not only encourages sufficient chewing to start off the digestive process, but you taste more of your food. Try to find all of the different flavours within your meal.

If you need to lose a few pounds, appreciation of the food you are chewing helps to quell the habit of eating more than you really need as it gives your body time to register the amount of food you have swallowed.

Starting the day calmly means that you are less likely to forget the important things that you need to take with you. There will be no last-minute panics. Your day will be organized, productive, and stimulating.

# Wake-up routine

Have you ever thrown your feet and calves into a cramp by stretching through to your toes just as you wake up in the morning? By stretching with awareness you can avoid this painful occurrence.

This routine is a very gentle but effective way of waking up your body. Begin before you get out of bed.

## NOTES AND SUGGESTIONS

Perform the movements slowly. Breathe in on each stretch and imagine the breath reaching deep within as it follows the stretch. When stretching your legs, be aware of any cramping reaction in your feet or calves and relax your body if you feel this happening.

Always continue breathing in as you tense your muscles and out as you relax.

### STRETCHING & STROKING

1. Lie on your back, with your arms above your head. Breathe in and stretch through to your elbows. Breathe out and straighten your arms. On the next breath continue the stretch to your wrists, then ease it out into your fingers. Breathe out into your fingers. Take your awareness back to your shoulders and, in one smooth movement, extend the stretch all the way up to your fingertips, following the ripple of muscles with your mind and your breath .

2. Take your awareness to the back of your neck and ease the stretch out again, following with your breath. This time move it up through your neck and scalp to the top of your head. Relax.

3. Go back to your neck and stretch all your arm and back muscles smoothly upward through your arms and downward to the tops of your legs without tensing your abdominals. Relax.

4. Breathe in and stretch all of the muscles down your front, rippling your abdominal muscles. Relax.

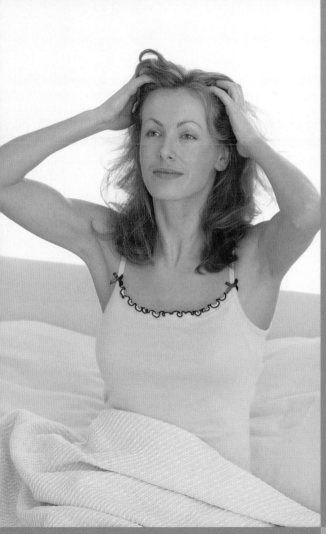

5. Take the stretch down your legs to your heels, stretching your body slowly and fully before taking the movement down to your toes. Keep the tension at your heels as you stretch your feet out. Hop out of bed and place your hands on top of your head. With your fingertips, stroke swiftly and lightly down your face and up the back of your head a few times. With loose fingers, scratch your whole head (see left).

6. Run your fingertips down the front of your body and up the sides as far toward your back as you can reach. Repeat a few times.

7. Run down the front of your legs to the toes and up the back of your legs. Repeat.

8. Stand still, inhaling, holding, and exhaling, each for a count of five. Repeat for ten cycles.

9. Relax, breathing normally.

# Tao Yinn and tapping routine

This routine is based in the tradition of the Tao Yinn. It fills your body with energy and clears your mind for the day ahead. You can do the complete routine using only open hands, fingertips, or closed fists, or you can vary it according to the area being worked. Stand with your body held loosely around a central thread that runs up from your feet, through your body, and out the crown of your head. Allow your breath to deepen and feel your heart rate slowing. Feel a connection with the earth. Inhale and pull the breath from far out in the universe into your body. Exhale and push the breath deep down into the earth. Repeat this for a few moments, until you feel you are at one with all. Try to keep your awareness of the connection open throughout the exercise.

1. *Start by placing your open hands flat on the top of your head. Close your fists and tap sharply over your head (see left) and down your face, working lightly over your eyes. Repeat three or four times, ending at your chin.*
2. *Beat down your neck, around the back of your neck, and up to the crown of your head.*
3. *Open your hands and gently slap them down over your face. Repeat this three or four times, ending with closed fists at the throat.*
4. *Beat with one fist across to the opposite shoulder (see right) and down the inside of your arm to your hand. Beat back up the outside of that arm and across your upper chest. Change hands and work in the same way across to the other side. Repeat this cycle three or four times.*
5. *Beat with both fists down your sternum (breastbone) to*

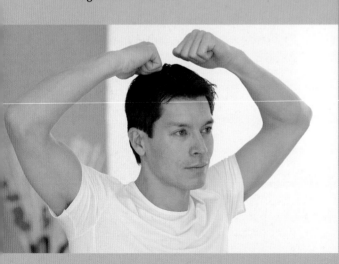

your abdomen. Then beat in a clockwise circle around your abdomen. Repeat this cycle three times.

6. Beat with both fists down your chest and abdomen to the tanden (two finger widths below your navel).

7. Work across to your back and, with the back of your fists, beat up as far as you can reach. Beat with one fist over your upper back and shoulder as far back as you can reach.

8. Change hands and work the other side of your upper back and shoulder. Each time you do this, try to extend your reach farther back.

9. Come back to your throat and repeat the cycle (steps 5 to 8) three or four times, ending at the tanden.

10. Beat with your fists down the front of your legs to your feet, then up the back of your legs to the top of your thighs. Repeat three or four

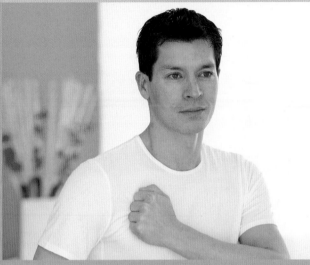

times, ending at your feet.

11. Allow your body to hang in this position for a few moments. Relax your whole body into this, but if you experience any cramp or discomfort come out of the hanging position.

12. Slowly straighten up, with your eyes closed, putting your awareness into the top of your head. Observe any sensations,

feelings, or emotions.

13. Move your awareness down into your chest and observe once again. Do this for three slow breaths.

14. Move your awareness into your abdomen, observe for three breaths. Put your awareness into your strong legs. Take three breaths.

15. Slowly open your eyes. Notice how alive, vibrant, but totally calm you feel.

# Breathing

Breathing keeps us alive, yet we don't think about it until we suddenly have to change our rhythm. It oxygenates our minds and bodies. It is necessary for cellular renewal and mental function, and releases the energy stored within our cells. It also detoxifies our bodies – about 80 per cent of the toxins in our system are eliminated through the breath. It can be used to alter our state of consciousness – hyperventilation and reduced oxygen supply to the brain can both affect our perception of reality.

Therapies such as rebirthing, which make use of breathing techniques to increase or decrease the oxygen levels in the brain, can affect ancient memory function, our emotions and feelings, and even our basic attitudes and behaviour patterns.

During the average day we use only our upper lungs, but if we do breathing exercises we use more of our lungs, enlarging their capacity by stretching the fibrous material of which they are made, enabling us to clear out any build-up of dead tissue and toxins, and draw in a greater oxygen supply.

Regular practice of breathing routines will also help with massage. As you move around your partner your breathing will adjust to your energy expenditure and there will be no puffing, jerking, or gasping, just smooth movement and rhythm.

Here is a modified form of an ancient Tantric breathing exercise that builds up and releases a high energy burst within us. It is sometimes known as the "violet breath" or "circular breath".

## TANTRIC BREATHING EXERCISE

*1. Stand straight, but relaxed, with your knees slightly bent and your eyes closed. Breathe deeply during the whole sequence. Observe your breathing. Feel your lungs working smoothly and efficiently.*

*2. Place the tip of your tongue just behind your upper front teeth. This closes the gap between the conceptual vessel, which runs from your lower lip, down the front of your body to the Hui Yin point just behind the genitals, and the governing vessel, which runs from the Hui Yin point, up the centre of your back, over the top of your head to your upper lip.*

*3. Put your awareness into the Hui Yin point. As you inhale, visualize your breath moving up the governing vessel, over the top of your head to meet the conceptual vessel at the tip of your tongue. As you exhale, visualize your breath moving*

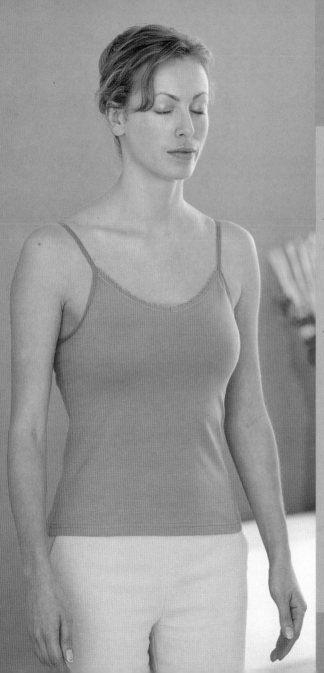

down the conceptual vessel to the Hui Yin point.
4. Follow this breath for three or four cycles, ending back at the Hui Yin point. As you end the last cycle on an out-breath, visualize a powerful energy moving with the breath. Pull this energy up through the governing vessel and down through the conceptual vessel.
5. Repeat this flow for ten breaths, then relax and open your eyes.

# Shower & bath massage

Combining massage with your shower or bath is very beneficial. Many therapies, such as Watsu and hydrotherapy, use the healing power of water, stretching, and massage to relieve various conditions. Stiff muscles and joints, sluggish blood and lymph circulation, poor elimination of toxins, constipation, and many more complaints can be helped through the use of hot and cold water sprays.

## IN THE SHOWER

If you wish to use essential oils with a shower it is best to massage the oil into your body first, relax, and have a cup of herbal tea. After about twenty minutes, have a shower. This gives the oils time to soak into your skin and they don't get washed away in the shower.

Hot water is initially stimulating and then relaxing. Cold water is invigorating and toning. Warm water makes you drowsy. Alternating the temperature of your shower revives your whole body.

To massage your body under a shower it is best to use a hand-held unit as this enables you to utilize the full force of the spray close to the showerhead. It will also help if you use a bath or shower seat so that you can more easily raise your feet to spray the soles.

## IN THE BATH

Bath massage is relaxing and stimulating, and certain forms of massage, such as underwater massage and massage in conjunction with mineral soaks, can treat a variety of conditions.

To get the best out of a massage in your bath,

### SHOWER MASSAGE

1. Run hot water over your whole body. Beginning with your feet, thoroughly massage all over each foot with strong kneading, joint rotations, squeezing, and pinching. Follow your massaging hand with the water spray.
2. Move slowly up to your calves, massaging with strong kneading and squeezing in an upward direction. This helps the natural flow of blood and lymph. Continue all the way up your legs, front, and back in the same manner, following the massage with the water.
3. Work up your abdomen, then work your chest, neck, face, and back.
4. Switch to cold water. Use a scrubbing brush in firm, circular movements, working from your feet to your head, taking care with the more delicate tissues.
5. Return to the hot water and, using your fingertips, scrub over your body with firm rotating movements.
6. Finish with an invigorating cold spray.

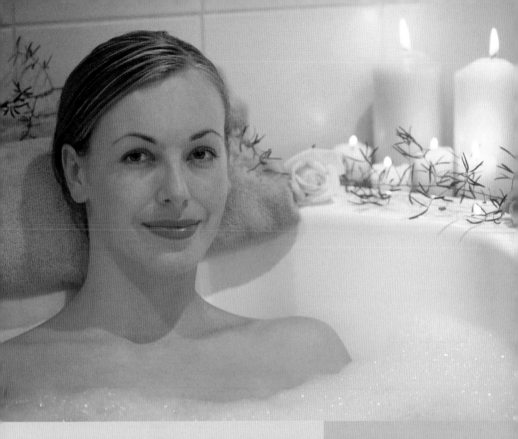

combine it with oils or place a small muslin bag filled with porridge oats under the running hot water tap. This is very good for skin complaints such as dry, sensitive skin, eczema, or psoriasis. You can use this with five drops of lavender and five drops of chamomile.

For a relaxing bath after a hard day use three drops of chamomile, three drops of geranium, and two drops of patchouli.

For an invigorating bath use three drops of rosemary and three drops of lemon.

### BATH MASSAGE
*Massage your body from the feet up, as in the shower sequence. This is incredibly relaxing but if you feel you need to wake up your body and mind, you could follow the bath with a refreshing cold shower.*

# Sweeping

Sweeping moves any surface energy congestion that has collected over your body, causing sluggishness.

### NOTES AND SUGGESTIONS

Your hands may feel as if they are coated in cotton wool. This feeling is caused by a build-up of static energy. Visualize a deep hole opening in the earth and vigorously flick off the coating into the hole.

Repeat all the movements in this sequence three to four times.

*1. Put both hands on your face and move them swiftly upward over your face and head, then down to the back of your neck (see left).*
*2. Place one hand on your opposite shoulder at the base of your neck and sweep it down to your fingertips. Repeat with the other hand.*
*3. Place both hands on your chest and sweep down the front of your body.*
*4. Put your hands as far up as you can reach on your back and sweep down.*
*5. Place both hands on the top of one leg and sweep down to your feet. Repeat with the other leg.*
*6. Stand relaxed, knees slightly bent, arms by your sides. Shake your head loosely from side to side.*
*7. Grasp the hair on the top of your head, close to the scalp, and shake it vigorously. Repeat with the hair at the sides and back of your head.*
*8. Drop your arms. Take several deep breaths, visualizing the air moving down to the soles of your feet on the in-breath and roaring up from your feet and out the top of your head on the out-breath. Do this for five to ten breaths.*

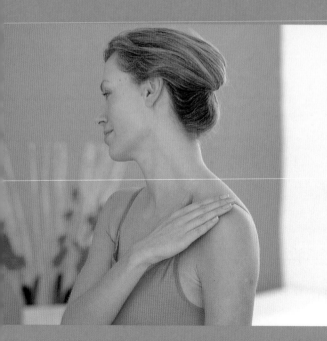

# Shaking

Shaking vibrates every cell in our bodies, forcing them to pull in oxygen and nutrients and squeeze out waste matter. It improves circulation and frees up your breathing. It also activates the release of energy within each cell, powering up your mind and body.

## NOTES AND SUGGESTIONS
The movement is swift and small. Imagine you are connected to a surging electrical current.

1. *Allow your breathing to relax. Put your awareness into the soles of your feet. Shake your feet, gently at first, then more vigorously. Bring the shaking up into your legs. Feel every cell of your feet and legs moving. Bring it up from your legs into your body. Feel all your internal organs shaking.*
2. *Take the shaking into your hands and arms, feeling the vibration travel from fingertips to shoulders.*
3. *Move the shaking into your neck and head, feeling the zinging vibrations.*
4. *Take your awareness back down to your feet and move it slowly up through your body, keeping in touch with the vibration of every cell. Try to identify and move with every cell.*
5. *As you reach your head, drop your awareness back down to your feet. Keep this cycle going for about five turns, then relax.*
6. *Allow the shaking to subside. Breathe in long, slow breaths. Don't try to do or be anything, just feel the existence of every cell in your body.*
7. *When you feel ready, bring yourself back to a state of full awareness.*

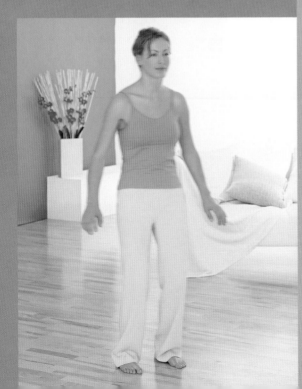

# Ailments and their pressure points

■ *Anxiety, panic attacks* If you are under pressure at work you may find that your levels of anxiety rise or you may even suffer a panic attack. To help in these situations place your fingertips on a pressure point at the centre of your sternum, CV17. Breathe slowly and deeply, and visualize a calming blue cloud around you. After a few moments you will feel your anxiety draining away. To maintain a calm and centred outlook on life it is worthwhile investing 15 to 20 minutes each day in a soothing massage and meditation, and taking regular exercise to boost your oxygen levels. You will find that recurrence of the attacks will decrease. H7, on the wrist, is also a good calming point.

■ *Backache* Emotional stress as well as poor posture can aggravate lower back problems. For quick relief, ask a partner or colleague to help. (Do not use this massage if the problem is a medical condition.) Sit on a stool with your elbows on your knees or straddle an armless chair, facing its back. Have your partner place their hands on your lower back, with the heels about two finger widths from your spine and their fingers angled at about 45 degrees. Ask them to lean in with all of their weight and 'walk' up and down your back, hand over hand, for a few moments. This will loosen any tension. There are also pressure points that you can use – B23, which are located just up from waist level and about two finger widths out from either side of the spine, and B47, which are about two finger widths to the outer sides of B23. They could be quite tender, so use them with care. Use fists, fingers, or thumbs to apply a firm pressure for a few moments.

■ *Breathing difficulties* There are several pressure points that will help relieve breathing problems. On your hand there are two, L9 and L10. These are near your thumbs. L9 is at the base of the inside of your thumb and L10 is about two finger widths up along the thumb bone. Briskly rub these points on both hands, for a few moments. Some breathing difficulties are caused by toxin build-up within your body. To help to move these, massage points B13, K27, and L1 regularly. B13 are situated two finger widths either side of the spine and one finger width below the level of the shoulder blades. K27 are in the hollow just below the collarbone and either side of your sternum. L1 are just inward from each shoulder joint and three finger widths below the sternum. As breathing problems can be triggered by emotional stress the treatment for anxiety can be beneficial.

■ *Colds* There are many pressure points around the face and head that will help drain a cold and clear the sinuses. GB20 are at the base of the skull and about two finger widths either side of the spine, in the dimply area. Strong massage here will quickly help to clear a cold. GV16, which is in the centre between the two GB20's, is a very good point for other symptoms such as headache and stiff necks. For the sinuses, apply pressure to B2, in the inner corner of the eyebrows. Pressure to the LI20 points either side of your nose, will also help your sinuses.

■ *Hangovers* You will need to encourage the body to move the toxins of alcohol and help the blood flow to the brain. Massage strongly into LI4, which is in the fleshy area between the thumb and first finger of each hand. The points for eye strain will help with headache; these are B2, ST3, and GV24.5, the latter of which is in the centre of the forehead. A gentle head massage may help but you may feel too delicate for this.

■ *Insomnia* A long leisurely bath with lavender oil, a cup of peppermint tea, a full body massage, or a head massage, concentrating on your upper back and neck, will help to release any physical and emotional problems that stop you getting a good night's sleep. You can also massage some of the anaesthetic points given in the general pain section (see p.42), especially LI4. Massaging the earlobes can also help to relax the mind.

■ *Stomach problems* As a preventive measure, regular massage on CV12, half-way between the navel and the base of the sternum is very useful, but avoid this point if you have just eaten or if you have high blood pressure or heart disease. About two finger widths below the navel is CV6 – massage this point if you are suffering from digestive upset, abdominal pain, or constipation.

*Refer to pp.16–19 and 42–3 in order to locate the various pressure points.*

■ *General pain* As well as massaging the painful area with thumb and palm rubbing, there are pressure points for the root cause of the pain. For the upper body, massage with strong rotations or continuous pressure on: point LI4, which is found in the fleshy area between the thumb and first finger of each hand; GV24.5, at the bridge of the nose between the eyes; GB20, at the base of the skull, two finger widths either side of the spine; and GV16, at the top of the spine where it meets the head. For lower body pain you can massage ST36, which is found about four finger widths below the kneecap and one finger width from the bone toward the outer area of the leg. If you press on this spot and move your foot you should feel a movement in the muscle. It can also feel quite painful under pressure. K3, on the inside of the ankle in the dimply area between the bone and the Achilles tendon, is another good pressure point, as is B60, which can be found on the outside of the ankle at the same level.

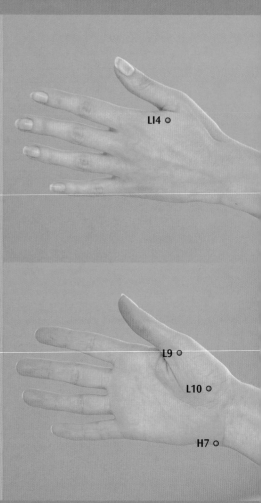

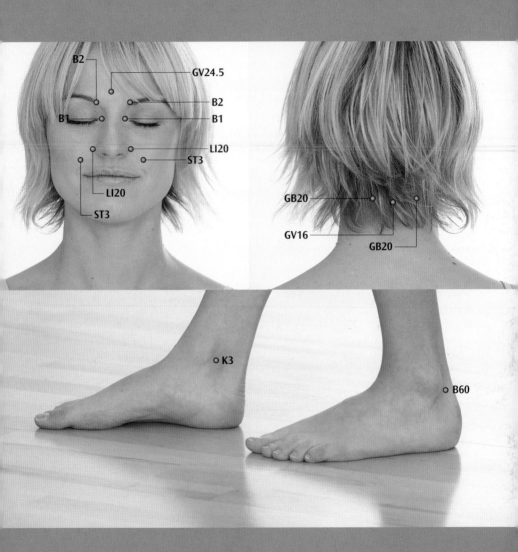

# Chakra meditation

I shall be using the term "chakra" as it is commonly understood, to mean an energy centre of the body and aura. There are many more chakras within the human energy system than the seven main ones that are usually worked. Tiny chakras are found throughout the body and aura. We are literally surrounded by hundreds of these minor energy centres, each of which is connected with every other chakra. In disciplines such as Shiatsu, which recognizes meridians with various tsubos (pressure points) along their lengths, many of these minor chakras are worked. Those who use energy healing systems also connect with the chakras within the auras to detect and treat the various disturbances that can cause ill health.

This chakra meditation is very energizing so it is a good idea to do it in the morning or at midday rather than in the evening. If you practise the sequence regularly you will find that it has a cumulative effect which will help to build your stamina, calm your mind, open your awareness, and develop your intuition. It will strengthen your healing powers and allow you to give more to your partner during massage without draining your own energy supplies. Allow yourself to be with the power of the light. It may feel strange at first – light-headedness and slight dizziness are normal reactions. If you wish you can do the meditation sitting down until you become used to the physical sensations that accompany it.

Your room should be comfortably warm and well aired, perhaps with a scented oil burning and low, soft music playing, or silence, if you prefer.

*1. Stand with your feet about shoulder-width apart, your knees flexible and slightly bent, and your arms hanging loosely by your sides. Breathe slowly and deeply, but without directing your breath at this stage.*

*2. Put your attention into the earth beneath your feet. Feel it as a living entity. Connect with the life of all things.*

*3. Move your awareness deep into the earth, to the fire energy of its centre. Feel that connection moving up through your body and out from the top of your head.*

*4. Slowly move your attention up through the air above you. Feel the connection between the earth and the universe.*

*5. Move your awareness to the farthest parts of the universe. You are now within a channel that leads from the centre of the earth out to the universe. Visualize the sun and the moon in a straight line with you in the channel between them.*

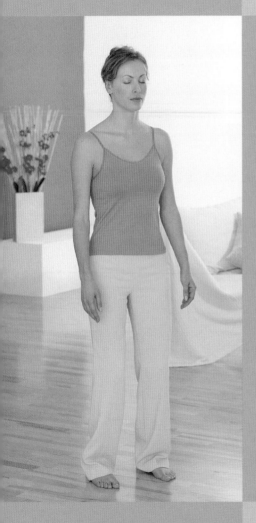

6. Breathe in – see a light coming from the universe to the sun.

Breathe out – feel the sun absorbing the light and growing brighter.

Breathe in – see the bright light moving from the sun to the moon.

Breathe out – feel the moon absorbing the light and growing brighter.

Breathe in – see the light moving from the moon to a point, a chakra, about one metre (3 feet) above your head. This is your transpersonal point.

Breathe out – feel this chakra glowing with a bright white light. You may now feel the power of the energy moving within your aura.

Breathe in – see the light enter the top of your head, your crown chakra.

Breathe out – feel your crown chakra absorbing the power and glowing with a violet light.

Breathe in – see the light move down into your third eye (brow) chakra.

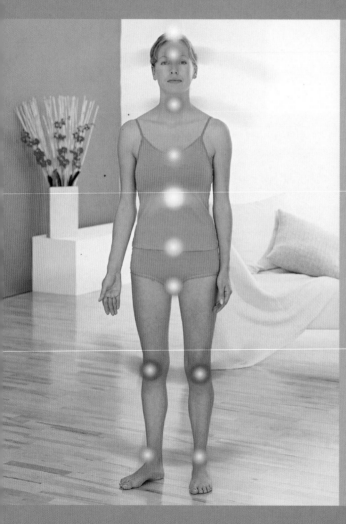

*Breathe out – feel your third eye chakra glowing with an indigo light.*
*Breathe in – see the light continue to move down to your throat chakra.*
*Breathe out – feel your throat chakra glowing with a soft blue light.*
*Breathe in – see the light branch out and move across your shoulders and down your arms, into your hands and palm chakras.*
*Breathe out – feel your arms and hands filling with a silver light. Open your hands. Feel your fingers extending down into the earth to open the channel and complete this connection.*
*Breathe in – see the light move down your body to your heart chakra.*
*Breathe out – feel your heart chakra glowing with a green light. (You may also have a sense of pink or turquoise with this chakra – some people have become aware of another chakra opening just above the heart chakra.*

*If you feel this, just allow the
light to fill the whole area of
your upper chest.)*
*Breathe in – see the light
move down to the solar
plexus chakra.*
*Breathe out – feel your
solar plexus glowing with
a yellow light.*
*Breathe in – see the light
move down to your sacral
chakra (hara).*
*Breathe out – feel your
sacral chakra glowing with
an orange light.*
*Breathe in – see the light
continue to move down to
your base chakra.*
*Breathe out – feel your base
chakra glowing with a
vibrant red light.*
*Breathe in – see the light
move down to your knees
(minor chakra).*
*Breathe out – feel your knees
glowing with a dark holly-
green light.*
*Breathe in – see the light
move down to your feet
(minor chakra).*
*Breathe out – feel your feet
glowing with a dark russet-
brown light.*

*Breathe in – see the light
move down to your earth
point (this is a minor chakra)
about one metre (3 feet)
below your feet.*
*Breathe out – feel this point
glowing with a black light
(the opposite and balance
to your transpersonal point).*
*Breathe in – see the light
move down to the centre
of the earth. Move your
attention back out to the
universe once more.*
*Breathe out – feel the light
streaming down from the
universe, through your
chakras, gathering all of
the colours as it goes. The
light moves down to the
centre of the earth.*
*Breathe in – see a fountain
of light spray out all around
you from the centre of the
earth, lighting up all of the
hundreds of chakras within
your aura as it moves in a
vast ball of light that
encompasses the universe
and all within it.*
*7. Continue breathing and
moving this energy ball from
the universe, down through*

*your body to the centre of
the earth and back to the
universe, lighting up and
strengthening your whole
being, for about seven slow,
smooth breaths.*
*8. Slowly, on the final out-
breath, ending far out in
the universe, start to close
down the column of light.
As you breathe in, feel the
light dimming. Close down
all of the chakras within
your aura.*
*Breathe evenly with long,
slow breaths.*
*9. Draw the light up the
column through each chakra
(don't tighten up at this
stage, the chakras need
some movement), closing
them gently like a flower at
evening until you reach your
transpersonal point, a metre
(3 feet) above your head.
Then gather all of the energy
and move it back down into
your sacral chakra.*
*10. Finally, gently close
your sacral chakra.
Allow your breathing to
return to normal and come
back to full awareness.*

CHAPTER THREE

# Massage on the move

The journey to and from your place of work can be a trying time. Crowded roads, buses, and trains create and hold high levels of aggressive energy. However, you could also see your journey as a little break between home and work where you can enjoy the changing scenery, listen to music, talk to people.

If you are driving use every stop, tailback, and snarl-up as an opportunity to refresh your levels of calm, and stretch your hands to ease out that tense grip. Shrug your shoulders and roll your head to ease tired neck muscles. A small cushion placed at your lower back will help to support you and make your sitting position more comfortable.

If you travel on crowded trains and buses, your legs and back may ache through inactivity, and if you are strap-hanging, your arms may also need some help to release any cramps. Moving your weight slightly every few moments will help your circulation and will slide muscle tissues over each other, releasing any build-up of toxins within the fibres.

If you travel in a closed vehicle, you keep breathing the same tired air, which will contain a higher than normal level of carbon dioxide and bacteria. The best way to combat these problems is to walk as far as you can during any journey. Park your car at a car park farther away than usual from your place of work, get on and off trains and buses at stops a little farther from work, enjoy the breeze in your hair, and feel a part of your surroundings. If you have to travel by plane, take regular walks up and down the aisles to clear your mind and body of the staleness, stress, and tension of travelling.

# The importance of breathing

Every thought we have influences every breath we take. In a tense or even exciting situation our brains and our bodies need more oxygen. This releases the energy that enables us to think faster and respond rapidly. As this function is more under the control of our autonomic nervous system than our conscious direction, it can easily move into overdrive.

Stress, fear, fun, or just physical exertion all trigger a similar response. We breathe more rapidly, our heart rate increases, and our bodies prepare for action. All of this pulls extra oxygen into our bloodstream, making it more alkaline. If this extra oxygen isn't used up it can cause physical problems such as dizziness, fainting, tingling and numbness in your scalp and hands, and even visual disturbances. This is the body's way of shutting down to reduce the rate at which oxygen is consumed. Your conscious mind interprets these symptoms as anxiety and panic, which is why even mildly stressful situations, such as those that arise every day when we are travelling, can induce what we consider to be irrational fears. At this point we need less oxygen and more carbon dioxide. Well-controlled breathing will maintain a good balance of carbon dioxide and oxygen in the bloodstream.

Doing a few breathing exercises before or during massage will help to oxygenate the muscles, thus releasing muscle tension during a relaxing massage. Good breath control also helps to release toxins and waste products within the muscle structure, which can then be carried away by the blood.

# Alternate nostril breathing

This technique calms the mind, reduces facial pain, clears the sinuses, and relaxes the jaw. It helps you to focus mentally and physically, facilitating concentration, and calms over-stimulating thoughts.

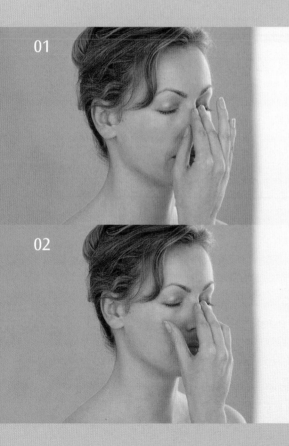

01

02

*1. Hold your right thumb against your right nostril to close it and, slowly, to a count of five, breathe in through your left nostril (01). Hold your breath for a count of five.*
*2. Release your right nostril and hold your left nostril closed with your finger (02). Breathe out for a slow count of five. Hold your breath for a count of five.*
*3. Repeat steps 1 and 2 about ten times, or more if you feel you need to. This will help to clear your head, reduce your anxieties, and provide a good supply of oxygen to your bloodstream.*

# Walking to work

Many people who work long hours can feel that they are missing out on life. Days come and go in a blur of meetings, decisions, dashing from one crisis to the next, and battling with confusion. While life is dancing all around them, they can feel very disconnected.

Walking to work, even in bad weather, can help to reconnect you, and it's a most enjoyable way to travel. You can breathe fresh air, get some refreshing exercise, and travel slowly enough to appreciate the changing seasons and all that is going on around you. If you live at some distance from your place of work, get off the bus a few stops before your destination and walk the rest of the way.

Walking with awareness can be used to give yourself an internal massage. By putting your awareness into your body and feeling exactly how your bones, muscles, tendons, and internal organs are moving, you can actively direct minute movements that stimulate a massaging of fibre on fibre. If you walk with awareness you can help your body to build up fitness, eliminate waste products, oxygenate tissues, increase flexibility, and relax your entire being.

Give yourself the time to really enjoy your walk. Allow time to make detours to new and interesting places, such as river banks, different market places, across fields, and through woodland. If you have to walk through streets, try different ways of reaching your destination – walk through a city park or along a canal bank. This can help you to see life fresh and new each day. Talk to people – even in the busy rush of morning there are interesting ideas to be explored, and seeing friends and making new ones helps to keep the channels of communication open.

While you walk, observe the ways you move your limbs, balance, and shift your weight as you take each step. Feel your back muscles – are they stooped? Change your posture, carry your weight high, imagine your whole weight as a ball above your head, and look around you instead of at the ground. This will help to rebalance and realign your whole body and pull energizing fresh air deep into your lungs.

Breathe deeply – even in a busy street, with passing traffic, deep breathing will help to clear your mind and remove toxins from your body. Over 80 per cent of detoxing happens through the breath. Good levels of oxygen are also necessary for the efficient release of energy within the body and for effective brain work.

You can also try a walking meditation. This is simply stilling your mind and being totally aware of moving one step at a time as you travel through space. Synchronize your breathing with your steps. Bring a smooth rhythm to all of your movements. Put your awareness into each tiny movement, but at the same time keep contact with everything that is going on around you. Even walking has its dangers.

Arriving at work after walking is very different from arriving after driving or travelling on a crowded train or bus. You feel more alive and ready for the day's challenges, rather than tired and headachy.

# Massage for travelling

## HEAD MASSAGE

Headaches are common travelling complaints. Low oxygenation, stale cabin air, immobility, and altitude can all adversely affect you. To help to restore the balance of pressure within your head, clear your sinuses, and help to ease tired eyes, try this pressure massage.

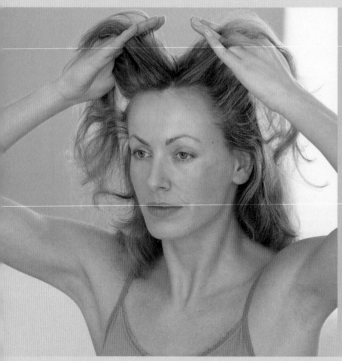

*1. Place your thumbs just under your jaw, by your ears, and drop the weight of your head on to them. Hold for a count of five and release.*
*2. Move your thumbs a finger width down your jaw in the direction of your chin and drop your head on to them again and hold. Repeat all along your jaw line.*
*3. Place the fingers of each hand under your cheekbones, so that your little fingers are either side of your nose.*
*4. Drop the weight of your head on to your fingers. Hold for a slow count of ten and release. Breathe slowly through your nose. Repeat this three times.*

## NECK MASSAGE

To ease an aching neck, hold your head with both hands and toss your head loosely from side to side. Try to take your head to its limit of movement. This should be a gentle action. Keep full control of the weight of your head with your hands at all times. Try to relax your neck and shoulders more each time your head moves.

1. *Place the fingers of both hands on the back of your neck, either side of your spine and running down the length of your neck vertebra.*
2. *With strong rotations work your fingers firmly into the muscles of the neck, for a count of five.*
3. *Move your fingers sideways by one finger width and again work firmly into your neck. Repeat twice more and then relax your neck.*
4. *Drop your head forward, swinging it slowly from side to side to loosen the muscles.*
5. *Hook your thumbs into the hollows located at both sides of the spine at the top of your neck.*
6. *Firmly push in an upward direction while slowly moving your head back on to your thumbs. Hold this position for a count of ten. Release and relax.*
7. *Rub the whole of the back of your neck firmly with your knuckles.*

5. *Close your eyes. Place your thumbs under your eyebrows either side of your nose. Drop the weight of your head on to your thumbs. Hold for a slow count of ten. Release, screw up your eyes, and hold for a count of ten. Repeat this three times.*
6. *Place all the fingers of both hands in a line along your hairline so that your little fingers are touching. Press firmly into your scalp and hold for a count of ten. Move your fingers about a finger width back toward the crown of your head and repeat the pressure.*
7. *Repeat the pressure in one finger width intervals until you have reached the crown of your head.*

8. *Place your fingers in a vertical line at the sides of your head, in line with your ears, and repeat the pressure massage backward until your fingers meet at the back of your head.*
9. *Run your fingers through the hair over the top of your head. Close your fingers up together so that you are holding a good handful of hair in each hand and pull firmly out from the scalp so that your hair is slowly running under tension through your fingers (see left). Repeat this pull in a perpendicular direction, all over your head.*

## SHOULDER MASSAGE

For shoulder aches, place your left hand on your right shoulder, just under your right ear, and grasp firmly (see below). Hold the pinch for a count of three. Move down your shoulder about a palm width and repeat. Repeat this along your other shoulder. There are some very powerful pressure points along your shoulders which may be painful, but it is very good to work them firmly. Do not use this technique over the middle of your shoulders, GB21, if you are pregnant.

*1. Raise your right arm above your head and take hold of the elbow with your left hand.*
*2. Drop your right hand down behind your head. Exert pressure with your left hand to extend the stretch and hold for about 20 seconds. Repeat on the other side.*
*3. Shrug your shoulders several times up and down and then backward and forward several times.*
*4. Raise both hands in the air. Cross them over and try to grasp as far down one arm as you can. While holding with one hand, try to creep the fingers of the other hand farther down the arm, then hold firmly. Then do the same with the other hand. Hold the final position for a count of five.*
*5. Relax.*

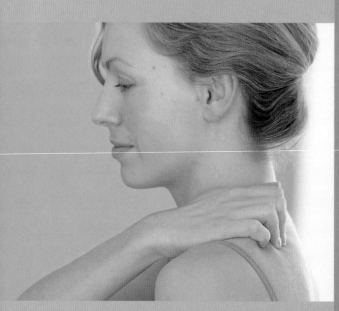

## ARM AND HAND MASSAGE

When you have finished the shoulder massage, move on down to your arms. Explore the movement of your wrists and hands in all directions.

Hold your wrists in the extreme positions for a count of ten for each movement, and release. Do the same with each of your fingers. This will loosen your wrists and hands and improve their flexibility.

*1. Grasp the top of your right arm with your left hand and firmly knead with your fingers and thumb down your arm and into your hand (01). Continue the kneading all over your hand (02).*
*2. When you reach the end of each finger, firmly pinch the fingertip and pull strongly, then shake vigorously. Repeat with the other arm and hand.*

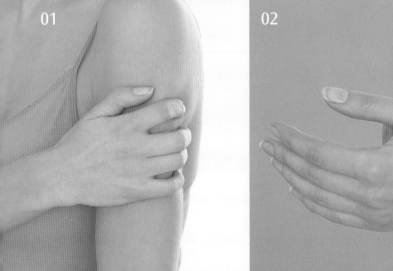

01

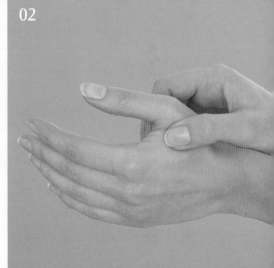

02

## ABDOMINAL MASSAGE

Travelling often causes stomach upsets. Strange food, tension, and the smell of diesel or aviation fuel can all trigger symptoms of nausea, constipation, and diarrhoea. To combat the smell of fuel a few drops of lavender and frankincense on a tissue or your clothing can help to disguise any unpleasantness and calm you.

### Stomach upsets:

Massage with rotations on points ST43 and ST44, which are on the top of your feet, just between your second and third toes (see pp.18–19). They are very close together so if you massage from between your toes to about one finger width below the base of your toes you will be working the correct area. Another two points are ST41, at the centre front of your ankle, and ST36, four finger widths below your kneecap, on the outer side of your leg.

### Other digestive disorders:

1. Using your fist, massage in gentle rotations from right to left across the whole of your abdominal area.
2. You can also use 'the wave'. Press with the heel of your right hand on the right side of your stomach and firmly slide across to the left side of your stomach.
3. Roll the pressure along your hand to your fingertips and, gently pressing in with your fingertips, pull your hand back across your stomach. Repeat this all over your stomach area.

### BACK MASSAGE

1. Make your hands into fists and hold the knuckles of each hand against your spine as low down your back as you can reach without discomfort.
2. Lean back slightly on to your hands so that you can feel a strong pressure against your spine. Massage into your back for a few moments.
3. Keeping your hands at the same level, move your fists out toward your sides about a palm width and lean back again. Follow this with massage. Repeat across the full width of your back.
4. Go back to your spine to a position about a palm width higher and repeat the leaning back and the massage. Try to raise the level of your fist twice more and repeat the massage. This will loosen an aching back and will also benefit your shoulder flexibility.

## LEG AND FOOT MASSAGE

To help avoid deep vein thrombosis (DVT) on long journeys you should start to massage your legs every 20 to 30 minutes from the beginning of your trip.

*1. Take your shoes off and use the heel of one foot to massage your other leg strongly, from the top of your foot up to your knee (01). Massage in an upward direction. You can also use your toes and upper foot to massage the back of your calves (02).*

*2. Then continue by using your hands to massage one leg at a time with a strong kneading action, working in an upward direction, to encourage blood flow back to the body.*

*3. Continue the kneading massage up over your thighs, working into all of the muscles in that area (03).*

*CAUTION*
*Do not work strongly if you suffer from varicose veins.*

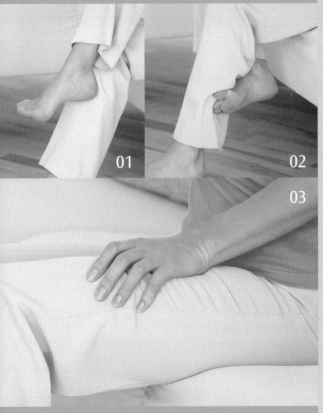

# CHAPTER FOUR

# Massage
# at work

It can be difficult to take more than a few moments out of your working day to use massage. The deep benefits of massage have much to do with allowing yourself to forget everything and let go. Even a few moments can be useful when you have a headache, tired eyes, or stiff muscles.

Having finally made it in to work through the rush hour you may already feel wound up, tense, stressed, and unable to face the day until you've had at least three cups of coffee. Resist this impulse.

Find a quiet corner. Bunch your hands into fists and vigorously rub your knuckles from the back of your head to the front, covering your whole head in sweep after energetic sweep. If you still feel tense, continue the knuckling down your neck, across your shoulders, down each arm in turn, down your front, and over your back.

There are some pressure points running down the length of your sternum (breastbone) that can help to clear your breathing if your chest feels tight. Press as hard as you can at the top of your sternum with your index and middle fingers. Hold for a count of ten. Move down about two finger widths and repeat until the end of the sternum.

Work one leg at a time with strong knuckling, using both fists massaging either side of your leg, down to your feet. Repeat over the other leg.

Now use your breath to re-energize your system quickly. Take deep, long, slow breaths. As you breathe in, feel the breath pulling strong invigorating energy up from the centre of the earth. As you breathe out, push this energy into every cell of your being. Continue this breathing cycle for 15 to 20 breaths. If you feel dizzy or light-headed, stop the deep breaths and breathe normally, but continue the visualization until you have completed at least 15 cycles.

# Meditation

After a rush hour journey to work you may well feel the need to rid yourself of the hassle of the trip before even trying to think of anything else you have to do.

This meditation connects you to the power of colour. You can begin on any colour of the spectrum. I find that yellow makes a good start. If you are feeling harassed you can move in the red direction, ending in the calming blues and greens. If you need an energy boost, move through the blues toward the reds. Here we shall move in the red direction. You can do this meditation standing or seated.

## NOTES AND SUGGESTIONS

Always visualize your colour moving toward you through a mist. As you breathe in, you will feel the colour on which you are meditating deepening. As this happens, feel every changing shade of the colour.

While you are doing the meditation imagine the healing energies working and you will bring the body's self-healing abilities into action. If you are giving a massage you will release the power of the universal healing energies; if you are receiving one you will activate your own healing process, thus increasing the effectiveness of the massage.

1. Close your eyes and imagine that you are surrounded by a golden-yellow egg-shaped mist.

2. Breathe in and feel the colour deepen at the outer edges of the mist.

3. Breathe out and feel the deeper colour moving toward you, filling you with a rich yellow glow.

4. Breathe in and feel the outer edges slowly turning to a clear orange. Be fully aware of this colour, taste it, smell it, feel its touch.

5. Breathe out and feel the colour moving toward you, filling you with an energizing rich orange glow.

6. Breathe in and feel the edges darken to red.

7. Breathe out and feel the deeper colour moving toward you, filling you with an energizing rich red glow.

8. Breathe in and feel the colour changing to a rich purple. Feel the healing purple colour moving toward you.

9. Breathe out and feel the colour moving through you,

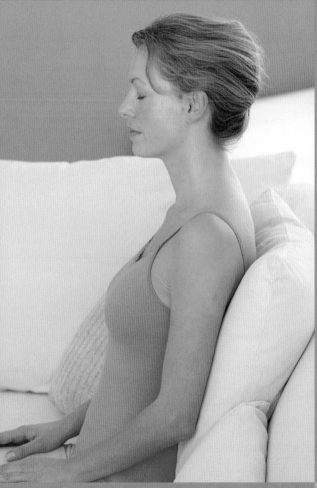

*filling you with an uplifting purple glow.*
*10. Breathe in and feel the colour changing to a rich royal blue.*
*11. Breathe out and feel the colour moving toward you, filling you with a deep, calming blue.*
*12. Breathe in and feel the colour lightening to a clear sky blue with wisps of turquoise and silver streaks.*
*13. Breathe out and feel the colour moving toward you, increasing your calmness.*
*14. Breathe in and feel the turquoise becoming greener.*
*15. Breathe out and feel the colour moving toward you. Feel your connection with all life growing.*
*16. Breathe in and feel streaks of light green/yellow moving in an energetic dance through you.*
*17. Forget your breathing and absorb the energy of this colour as you return to full awareness. Try to carry this feeling of a cool, bright spring day with you all day.*

# Coffee break massage

During your coffee break you can refresh your aching shoulders, arms, and hands. This will also help to ward off any tension headaches as it will loosen your upper back muscles. As your hands and arms contain many meridians, you can give your body a tone-up with a little hand and arm massage. Stretching your hands during your coffee break can help to ease any aches and improve their flexibility.

There are several channels running along both the outer and inner areas of your arms, from your fingertips to your upper body. These can be massaged to tone and stimulate not just the muscles and tendons of your arms but also your organs. While massaging your arm, breathe deeply and visualize a warmth moving down into the top of your head, through your body to your hara (lower abdomen), then back up into your arms. Try to see this cycle as a continuous, calming flow of energy.

**NOTES AND SUGGESTIONS**
TH4 is on the triple heater channel (see pp.16–17) and is very good for wrist pain. The triple heater is not really a specific organ, but a collection of organs that includes your lungs, and your digestive and elimination systems. Working this channel, which runs along your arm from the back of your ring finger up the length of the outside of your arm, can help with any abdominal and lower back pain.

Your middle finger carries the heart protector or pericardium channel, and massaging this point will help to ease any emotional stress, tightness in your chest, and indigestion.

The index finger holds the large intestine channel on its outside and massaging this will help with any abdominal problems such as flatulence, constipation, and diarrhoea.

Your thumb contains the lung channel, which runs up the inside of your hand and arm. L9, on the inside of your wrist, just below your thumb, and L10, located about two finger widths above L9 on your thumb, are very good points to massage if you are experiencing breathing problems (see pp.18–19 and p.42).

H7 is a point on the heart channel (see p.42). Working along both the heart channel and the small intestine channel will help to calm you, boost your energy, and clear your head.

The final stretch (see step 11, p.67) is very good if you have ever broken your hand or wrist as it will help you to regain complete flexibility.

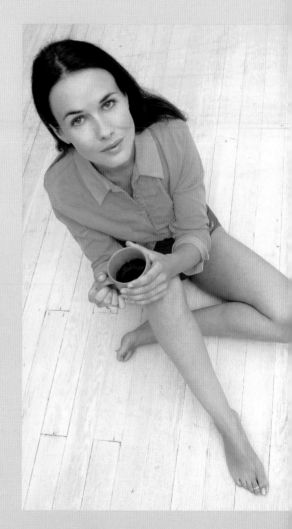

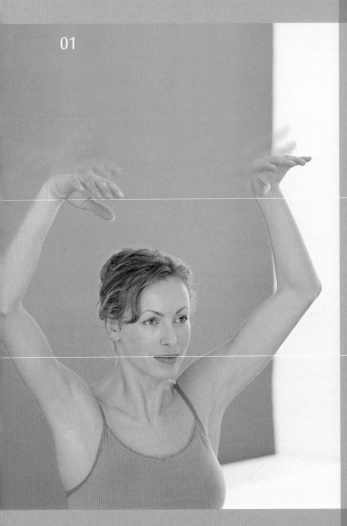

01

1. Hold your hands above your head for 20–30 seconds. Vigorously shake your fingers while they are still in the air (01). Shake your hands, then your arms, then your shoulders, moving them up and down, back and forth. This will boost the circulation in your hands and arms.

2. Lower the hands and grip one little finger with the thumb and fingers of your other hand, thumb on the top and fingers underneath. With strong pinching and kneading movements, work your way slowly along the outer edge of your hand.

At your wrist, spend a few moments massaging strongly into H7, just where the bones of your little finger meet the bones of your forearm (02). Move along your forearm up to your shoulder (03).

*3. Take hold of your ring finger and pinch and knead back along its length. Continue until you reach the joining of the finger bones with the forearm bones and here work with strong thumb rotations into TH4 (see pp. 16–17).*
*4. Repeat on your other arm.*
*5. Put your hands together and raise your elbows so that your forearms are at right angles to your hands.*
*6. Rotate your hands as far as they can go, away from your body. Hold that position for a count of ten.*
*7. Rotate your hands toward your body, as far as they can go, and again hold for a count of ten.*
*8. Come back to the centre and, while keeping the heels of your hands together, turn your fingertips toward you and push the heels of your hands away from you. Hold for a count of ten.*

*9. Come back to the centre. Push your left hand over to the left with your right hand. Make sure your hands make contact all the way down. Hold for a count of ten.*
*10. Come back to the centre and use your left hand to push your right hand over toward the right. Hold for a count of ten.*
*11. Lean your elbows on the desk and hold one hand with its palm toward you. Take hold of your little finger with your other hand and drop it back so that you are stretching your little finger back as far as it will go. Don't force the stretch, just allow the weight of your hand to move your finger backward. Hold for a count of ten. Repeat with the rest of your fingers and thumbs.*

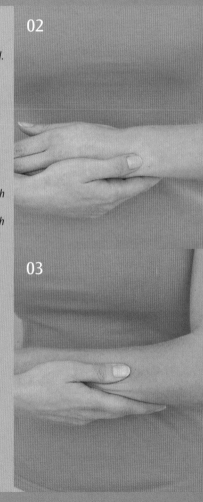

02

03

# Stretching, neck loosening

This is a full body workout which releases waste matter from the system, lubricates the joints, strengthens the muscles, and stretches the tendons. Since every cell in the body renews itself every few weeks, we can accumulate a great deal of waste matter through cellular degeneration and renewal. Inactivity, stress, tension, emotional problems, depression, illness, injury, and self-indulgence also deposit their own rubbish.

In an ideal world we would have perfect bodies, able to renew and refresh every cell without any problems. However, we don't get enough exercise, and we don't eat and drink only that which is good for our minds and bodies. Our thoughts are not based on that which brings good health and well-being to ourselves and our society. We enjoy danger, stress, and excitement. We have problems with relationships which wind us up and drop us from great emotional heights. In general, we treat ourselves very badly. This particularly affects the large muscles of our shoulders and neck. Mental stress immediately creates tension here, which can build up day after day to cause problems with pain and immobility – frozen shoulder, stiff neck, and tired, aching head and arms

Ideally, we should take on board only that which we need and will be of benefit to us. We need to produce energy to allow our minds to work, our bodies to move, and our spirits to create and enjoy. The process of energy production is based in combustion. Oxygen and calories in our food and drink burn to produce energy. This also produces waste matter. The exchange of food for waste products within our blood and lymph fluids should be able to rid our bodies of this waste. However, we tend to habitually abuse our bodies and overload our systems, and – over years – the waste products produced by these abuses and excesses, which our circulatory systems can't disburse, build up within our tissues, causing deposits that can affect our health. These deposits start as a coagulation, move on into a heavier gelatinous substance, and finally harden into a crystalline crust, which can eventually calcify and seriously injure our joints and under-used muscles.

This is where stretching and deep breathing exercises can help. When we stretch, the fibres within our muscles slide over each other. As these fibres slide, constant movement produces a pumping action, which breaks up any deposits within our muscles so that blood and lymph fluid can dissolve and carry away the refuse. Stretching to the fullest extent of our reach works deeply into these fibres, digging out old deposits. Aided by massage, you can go even farther. By breaking down hard-to-dissolve substances and squeezing and massaging them out of the fibres you can shift years of waste build-up, so helping to renew and regenerate your whole being. You feel calmer as your body relaxes into a healthy rhythm, without the strain and stress of having to work overtime trying to maintain a seized-up and clogged system.

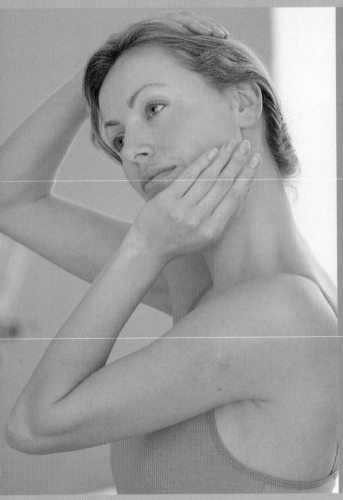

1. Stand with your feet about shoulder-width apart. Raise your arms and reach upward as far as you can. Breathe in deeply and out fully, and increase the stretch. Relax one arm but do not let it drop. Breathe in deeply and out fully and increase the stretch in the other arm.

2. Relax this arm and stretch your other arm. Breathe in deeply and out fully and increase the stretch.

3. Reach up with both arms. Breathe in and, as you let your breath go out, drop forward from your waist and allow your upper body to hang down loosely from your waist for a few slow breaths.

4. Feel the tension gradually draining out of your upper body. Start to swing gently from right to left. Don't force anything, just flop and swing for a count of 20–30. If you feel at all uncomfortable come out of the stretch, but each time you do the exercise, aim to extend your hanging count up to 60.

5. Stand up and stretch your arms out to the sides. Move one arm straight up above your head and allow it to bend at the elbow to drop the hand down behind your head. Swing the other hand up behind your back to meet it. If you can, clasp your fingers. Grip with your fingers as tightly as you can for a count of ten.

6. Release the tension, and then grip again. Repeat three or four times. Change your arms over, so that they are in the opposite position and repeat the stretch.

7. Sit down, allowing your arms to hang by your sides. Raise your shoulders until they meet your ears. Hold for a count of five, then drop them. Repeat this a few times until you can feel that your neck is holding some tension. On the last raise allow your head to drop to one side and, as you lower your shoulders, allow your head to be lowered on to one shoulder.

8. Raise both shoulders. At the top of the movement centre your head, then drop it on to the other shoulder.

9. Lower your shoulders and carry your head down with them. Repeat five times on each side.

10. Drop your head on to your chest. Clasp your hands behind your neck and pull your head farther down. Resist the pull of your arms by tensing your neck. Hold the pull for a count of ten.

11. Release and repeat the neck pull about 5 times or as many times as you can manage without feeling any discomfort or strain. While you have your hands behind your head and your head down, ask a colleague to pull up on your elbows for a few moments.

12. Come out of the stretch. Place your right hand on your neck, just under your left ear. With strong rotation, massage in a line across your shoulder. There are some quite painful spots here which respond well to strong massage. Work back and forth along this line for a few moments, then change hands and repeat along the opposite shoulder.

13. Hold the top left side of your head with your right hand (see left) and place the heel of your left hand on the right side of your chin. Pull gently with your right hand and push with your left, twisting your head round to the left. Hold for a count of 30. Release, bringing your head back to centre. Repeat on the other side.

# Dealing with indigestion

Working lunches, stress, and eating on the go can cause your stomach to rebel. For abdominal pains you will need to calm your mind and internal organs to allow them to release their tension.

1. Stand with your hands placed on your abdomen, just below your navel (tanden; see right). Take some deep slow breaths. On the in-breath, visualize a cool light, pale spring green or sky blue, moving into your body with your breath. On the out-breath, visualize this cooling, healing light filling your abdomen.
2. On the next in-breath, draw more of the cooling light into your abdomen, absorbing the pain and discomfort. On the next out-breath, push this light down your legs and out through the soles of your feet.

Continue breathing in this way as you slowly start to massage your stomach.
3. Place the heel of your right hand just under your ribcage on the right hand side. Press in firmly with the heel of your hand and slowly slide it across to the left side of your abdomen. Repeat this four or five times.
4. Move your right hand down about a hand width and repeat the massage.
5. Move your hand down once more and repeat again.
6. Place your left hand on your solar plexus. Hold the thumb and first three fingers of your right hand in a claw,

similar to the tiger's claw (see pp.98–9) but slightly tighter, with approximately 1 cm (1⁄2 in) distance between each finger.
7. Now starting on the right hand side of your abdomen, massage with small, firm, clockwise rotations, for about four or five rotations on each position. Work slowly, with the intention of dissolving the pain. Cover the whole of your abdomen with these rotations, moving from right to left.

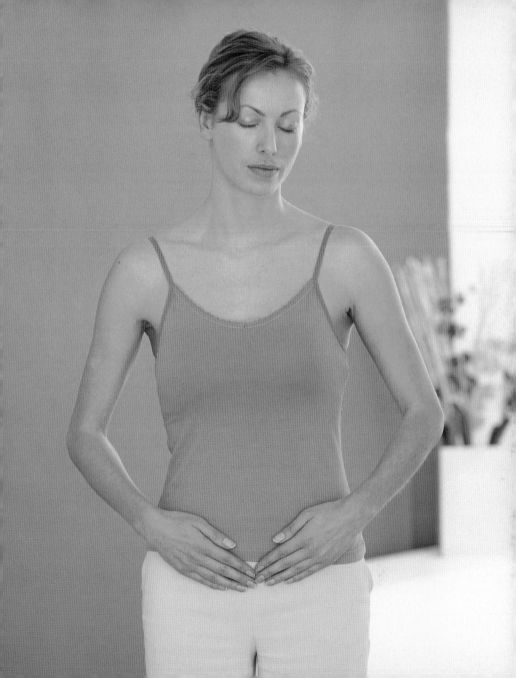

# Arm swinging

If after working for hours your arms and shoulders ache, your brain refuses to cooperate, and your legs feel as if they've collapsed into your feet, you can revive yourself with a simple meditation and swinging routine. You may be surprised how little time it takes to rejuvenate with this routine.

Arm swinging is one of the traditional warm-up exercises that therapists use before starting work for the day. It warms up the muscles, relaxes the mind, and clears the energy channels, which is why it is useful as a limbering-up exercise before massage.

*1. Stand with your feet about shoulder width apart and allow the weight of your head, neck, and shoulders to slide down your arms and out through your hands. Close your eyes if you wish, and feel all of the stress and tension in your upper body dripping from your fingertips down into the earth.*
*2. Slowly, pivoting your body around your waist, start to swing your arms. Allow them to move freely from your shoulders (see right).*
*3. Swing as far left as you can. Then, without breaking the rhythm, swing to the*

*right as far as you can. Allow your hands to flop at the ends of your wrists. Keep the whole movement loose and free-flowing. Swing back and forth. Forget time. Forget everything but the feeling of dead weights at the end of your arms, slapping against your body when they land. Swing back and forth. Keep the rhythm slow and even. Breathe with the rhythm. Inhale and swing one way. Exhale and swing the other way. Keep your eyes closed and allow the swing to become automatic, just allow it to simply happen.*

*4. Breathe in. Swing, visualize a light coming into the top of your head, flowing down to your waist.*
*5. Breathe out. Swing, see this light moving down and out of your feet, carrying all your tiredness with it. See it moving deep into the earth. Keep this pumping action going at a slow, steady pace. If outside problems start to intrude, just observe them, watch them flow past your mind as if on a TV screen. They are not part of you at this moment. Let them go. Feel yourself within a great pillar of light, steadily filling*

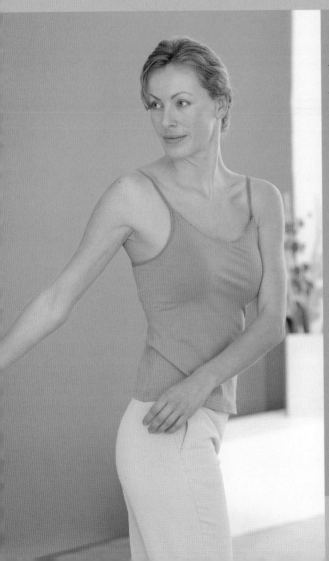

you up with energy.

6. Breathe in, feel your head filling with light.

7. Breathe out, feel the light flowing down your body, energizing and renewing your whole being.

On the in breath, slowly draw more and more energy into your body and mind. On the out breath, feel every last drop of tiredness leaving your body.

8. Feel the energy build with every breath, every swing. Remember to forget. See only yourself within this pillar of light. Physically connect with the light. If you feel your pace increasing slowly bring it back to a steady, comfortable swing. Be aware of the gentle slap of your hands against your body. Continue for as long as you wish. When you are ready, allow your hands to drop naturally by your sides. Take a few deep breaths and come back to full awareness.

# Clearing your head

Heavy headaches, poor concentration, and eye strain often occur in the mid-afternoon, especially if you have spent hours working at a computer. Poor posture, shallow breathing, telephones, glaring computer screens, and electrical equipment that produces a build-up of static negativity around us cause a variety of minor health problems every day. To combat these it is worthwhile taking a few moments now and again to move stiff muscles, re-oxygenate the brain and body, and rest tired eyes. It can also be helpful to keep a quartz crystal by your computer to help absorb static and to rebalance the surrounding energy.

If you can, move away from your computer or, better still, try to take a brisk walk outside of the building to get some air that has not been fed through an air-conditioning system, if only for a couple of minutes.

## HEADACHE AND EYE STRAIN

*1. Taking both hands, reach as far as you can behind your head and down your back. Then strongly massage into your upper back on either side of your spine for about a minute.*
*2. Move your hands up to your neck and repeat as strongly as you can. The points to use are the two B10 on the back of the neck.*
*3. Hook your thumbs into the hollows either side of your neck just as it joins your head. Press in an upward direction while leaning your head back against your thumbs. Hold this position for as long as possible – for at least 30 seconds.*
*4. Slide all four fingers of both hands to the back of your neck at the base of your skull and press inward and upward with your fingertips. Lean back into this and hold for 30 seconds. This covers GB20 and GV16.*
*5. Place the heels of your hands either side of the back of your head, level with your crown, spacing your hands*

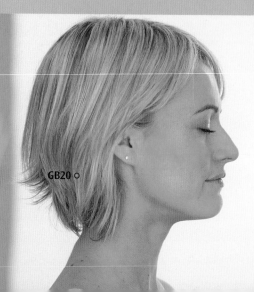

GB20 ○

so that you can just interlock your fingers over the top of your head. Now squeeze strongly with the heels of your hands in an upward direction. Hold for about 30 seconds. Release, move your hands midway toward the temples and repeat the squeeze. Move again so that the heels of your hands are against your temples and squeeze and hold again.

6. Place the palms of your hands over your eyes and relax into this position for three or four minutes. Press with your thumbs into the inner corners of your eyebrows, B2, for 30 seconds. Another good point is GV24.5 at the bridge of your nose between your eyes.

### CONCENTRATION LOSS

1. Hold point GV26, just under your nose and above your two front teeth, and GB20, which you can find by running your fingers up either side of your head, just behind your ears, till they meet on the top of your head. Hold these points at the same time, with a firm pressure, while taking deep breaths. Visualize your breath moving down to your abdomen and back up through the top of your head. Do this for ten breaths.

2. Relax and repeat twice, taking breaks between each count of ten so that you do not cause dizziness.

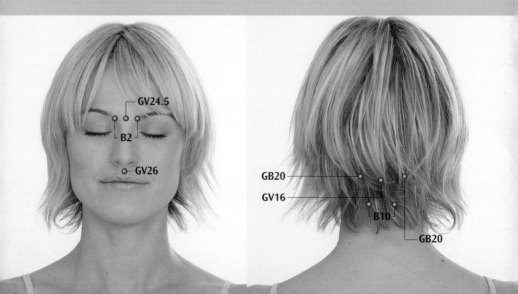

# CHAPTER FIVE

# Relaxing with head massage

It's the end of the day. You're home, warm, comfortable, and at peace? No? More often than not you'll have hot, swollen feet, an aching lower back, a muzzy head, a stiff neck, and more. This is because our bodies take quite a lot of punishment during an average day, causing us to feel less than well.

True relaxation can allow our bodies and minds to refresh themselves. When you arrive home it is worth taking time to make a conscious effort to break the connection with the day and its problems.

Lie flat on your back with your feet higher than your head for 20–30 minutes to enable the discs in your spine to re-inflate.

While you are lying there you can also help your head and body by palming. Place your hands on top of your head and feel their warmth. Observe this warmth, feel it penetrating your scalp and your brain. Breathe slowly and deeply. Feel your breath drawing the heat into your head. Take about three to five minutes in this position.

Move your hands to your face. Hold your palms lightly over your eyes and again feel the warmth of your hands. Relax all the tiny muscles around your eyes. Allow your face to dissolve. Breathe the warmth into your face.

After three to five minutes move your hands to your ears and feel the warmth in your ears. Allow your jaw to loosen. Feel your breath filling your whole head.

Move one hand over your heart and place the other over the tanden (lower abdomen). Deepen your breathing. Feel the in-breath moving down through your body to the tanden and the out-breath rising up through your body to your heart. Feel the warmth from your hands filling your whole body while you breathe. Try to keep this cycle going for the rest of the time you are lying down.

# Head massage: setting the scene

Regular head massage not only benefits you by relaxing and loosening your shoulders, neck, and head but it also has a cumulative effect on your mental and emotional state. It can fire up your creativity. If you are struggling with a problem try this simple way of finding a solution. Condense the problem to a concise sentence. Repeat this to yourself three times, just before you have a head massage. Then forget it. Relax, enjoy your massage and by the time you have finished you will find that ideas will be pouring into your head. Don't try to make anything happen, just allow the process to run.

The techniques in this chapter have been taken from Indian head massage, Shiatsu, holistic massage, and others. They are gentle, releasing treatments, which are great for headache, stuffiness, stiff neck and shoulders, and have many other benefits. There are many pressure points within your face and head that connect with the whole of your being. These can be stimulated by stroking or toning, or if excess energy is the problem, as in the case of an inability to concentrate or focus, they can disperse this excess and calm your mind. Head massage also affects the pulsing rhythms of the cerebrospinal fluid which transmits healing around the body. This fluid runs up and down the spine and around the brain at a regular twelve cycles per minute carrying messages about the health and well-being of your whole system from the body to the brain and back again.

**A COOL HEAD**
*In a calm, relaxed frame of mind tensions within your body will dissolve. Head massage is a wonderful way to achieve this state.*

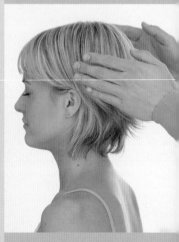

# Back massage: heel of hand rotations

Every time your brain works fast, even if you are just watching an exciting film, the muscles in your back tense for action. In the average day this tension can build up to become an almost permanent state. Massaging strongly into the back muscles encourages these muscles to release this tension. Working with one arm supporting your partner allows them to feel safe and comfortable, allowing their mind as well as their body to relax and let go.

## NOTES AND SUGGESTIONS
The pressure you use should be quite strong, but should not cause any pain.

*1. Move to your partner's side so that you can provide support with your arm across the chest.*
*2. Place the heel of your other hand about two finger widths away from the far side of the spine, at shoulder level (see left).*
*3. Now lean strongly into the back as you rotate for a count of five with the heel of your hand on the spot.*
*4. Move about three finger widths out toward the shoulder and repeat the movement.*
*5. Do this until you reach the shoulder, then come back to the centre. Move your hand about a palm's width down the back and repeat the rotations across to the side.*
*6. Cover the side with rotations, then change sides so that you can work on the rest of the back.*

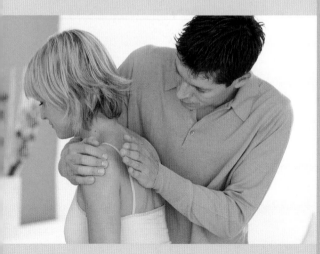

# Shoulder/arm pinch

This massage is very good for loosening up the back of
your neck and the large muscles of your shoulders and
your upper arms, which take most of the strain when
you are putting in long hours at a computer.

*1. Stand behind your partner
and grasp the shoulders,
either side of the neck. By
pushing down with the heel
of your hand and pulling
with your fingers, pinch
(don't nip) the flesh of the
shoulders in a forward,
rolling motion (01). The heels
of your hands should slide
toward your fingertips.
2. Move your hands about a
palm's width out across the
shoulders and repeat. You
are now moving into a
bonier area which could be
painful, so be guided by how
your partner feels about this.
3. Do the same movements
down the arms to the hands,
or as far as you can
comfortably reach (02). If you
can't do both shoulders and
arms together, just do them
one at a time, or substitute
a wringing action for the
pinch, which will also move
the fibres of the muscles.*

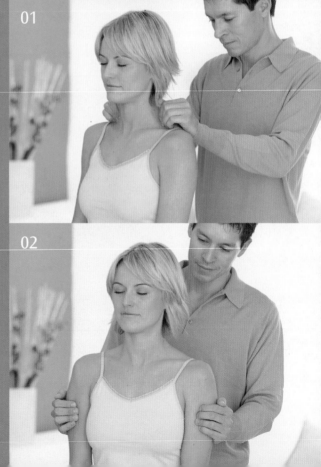

01

02

# Elbow rotations

This intensive massage is very good for releasing stiff necks and shoulders, improving the flexibility of the neck so that you can turn to look behind you more easily, which is particularly useful when driving a car.

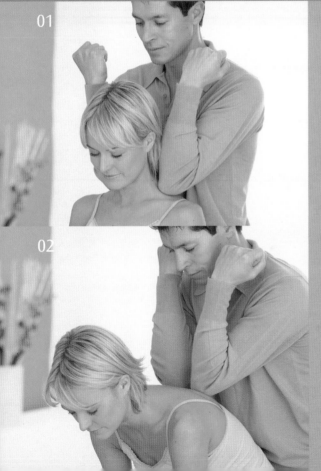

01

02

*1. Stand behind your seated partner and place your elbows, with your palms facing up, on the shoulders, close to either side of the neck. Have your forearms stretched out in front of you.*
*2. Close your fists and lean your body weight gently on to your elbows. Bring your fists up toward you, slowly (01). The closer you bring your fists toward you, the sharper your elbows will become and the stronger the pressure will be.*
*3. In this position, rotate your elbows smoothly for a count of five.*
*4. Relax and move your elbows out about three finger widths toward the arms and repeat, until you have worked the whole of the shoulders.*
*5. Repeat this movement by working your way down the back as far as you can (02).*

# Neck workout and still points

Many headaches, eye strain, and facial aches start around the neck area. This massage not only releases your immediate pains and stiffness, it can also, if used regularly, greatly reduce the effects of migraine, realign your head/neck balance, so easing any long held postural problems, and it can also help to alleviate tension-related tinnitus. The still points (GB20) are very useful for draining a cold. If you feel sniffly, headachy, or just fuzzy, you can massage by rotating with your finger and thumb on these points for a few moments every half hour or so. Your cold should rapidly work its way out of your system. You can use this technique as a self-treatment.

*CAUTION*
■ *Do not use this massage on anyone with a medical neck condition.*

*1. Still standing behind your partner, hold the forehead so that the head can drop forward slightly. With four fingers of the other hand, and starting about a finger's width from the spine, with your fingers running down the length of the vertebrae of the neck, gently rotate your fingers for a count of ten. This movement should be slow and very flowing. Repeat the movement two or three times, working your fingers out away from the spine in a circular spiral.*
*2. Change hands and repeat on the other side of the neck.*
*3. When you have completed both sides, place your thumb and first finger on either side of the spine, close to the head, in the dimply areas where the vertebrae meet the skull (see left). Press strongly in an upward direction into these still points for a count of five, then relax.*

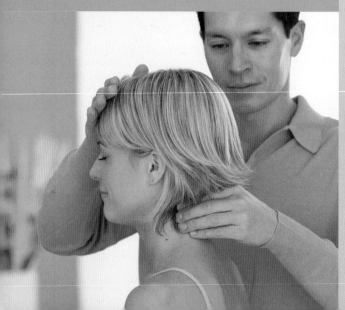

# Head scratching/ Hair pulling

Scratching is a very enlivening technique which helps to clear the mind.

Hair pulling can be used in conjunction with rotations (see p.86) or pressure (see p.87), to ease headaches, as it moves any stagnant and blocked energy in the head. It works in the opposite way to rotations by pulling the scalp away from the skull. It helps to release pressure imbalances in your head. It also helps to strengthen your hair roots and can regulate the flow of oils in your hair, easing problems of excessive grease or dryness in the hair and scalp. You can use hair pulling as a self-treatment.

## NOTES AND SUGGESTIONS

Keeping your fingernails in line while scratching will ensure that you do not snag the scalp.

### HEAD SCRATCHING

*You can do this with both hands or just one, with the other supporting your partner's forehead. Hold your hand(s) with the fingers curled so that your fingernails are in line with each other and scratch with a rapid, loose sideways action all over the head.*

### HAIR PULLING

*1. Starting with both hands at the back of your partner's head, run your hands up into the hair with your fingers spread open until you have a handful.*
*2. Close your fingers on the hair and, keeping a firm hold on the hair, pull your hands away from your partner's head in a perpendicular direction, allowing the hair to slide through your fingers (see left). Do this until you have covered the whole head.*

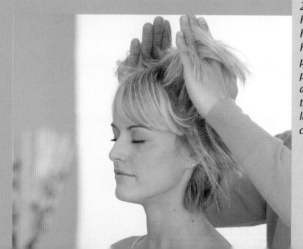

# Hair stroking/ combing, rotations

Hair stroking or combing is a gentle, calming technique and is one of the few head massage strokes that can safely be used for cancer sufferers, the very young, the elderly, and those suffering from bone diseases. It releases stress and tension, gently stimulates the hair and scalp, eases depression, and can help in cases of insomnia and hyperactivity.

Rotations disperse any excess energy within the meridians of the head. You can use both techniques as self-treatment.

## NOTES AND SUGGESTIONS

If your partner has long hair you may have to work in stages. If the hair is very short, open your fingers wide and, with a little pressure at the fingertips, start at the nape of the neck, following the same path as before.

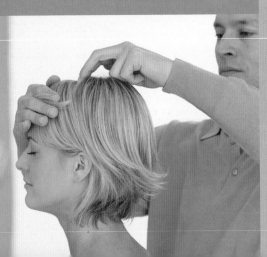

### STROKING/COMBING

*1. Still standing behind your partner, run both hands up into their hair.*
*2. Work with open fingers from the back of the neck to the forehead.*
*3. When you reach the hairline, comb your fingers through the hair, bringing your hands toward you. Then move your fingers up through the hair from the sides, starting just above the ears, up to the top of the head (see below left). Comb back through to the ears.*

### ROTATIONS

*1. Hold your partner's forehead with one hand so that they can bend forward slightly.*
*2. With two fingers of your other hand, start at the centre of the hairline, working in small rotations back to the nape of the neck.*
*3. Return to the front of the head to a position two finger widths to the side of your first line. Continue along a line parallel to the first. Repeat, moving two finger widths to the side for each new line, until you reach the ear. Repeat on the other side of the head.*

# Head shake, pressure

## HEAD SHAKE
*Run both hands into the hair and over the top of the head. When you have collected a handful, hold firmly and lightly shake the scalp back and forth (see below left). Don't pull hard, just enough to move the scalp.*

'Head shake' loosens the scalp and stimulates a good blood and nutrient flow to the roots of the hair. It also strengthens the root system which can help in cases of hair loss. As you get used to this technique you can work more vigorously. Head shake is very effective as a self-treatment.

Pressure is a very still technique, useful for toning any low energy areas in the meridians in the head, which can help your whole body and mind to achieve good health and well-being. In therapies such as Shiatsu, calming techniques like these are the opposite of the more vigorous, rotating moves. They help to maintain the overall balance and energy flow within the meridians by allowing them to absorb healing energy. On a physical level pressure can help to stabilize any imbalances within the flow of the fluids around the brain and release pain and tension in stressed muscles. You can use this technique as a self-treatment.

## PRESSURE
*1. Hold your partner's forehead with one hand. With two fingers of your other hand, start at the centre of the hairline and exert a firm pressure for a count of ten.*

*2. Release and move about two finger widths back and repeat the pressure. Continue until you reach the base of the neck and finish the line by pressing upward into the base of the skull.*

*3. Go back to the hairline and move two finger widths to one side. You are following the same lines as in rotations. Now repeat the pressure along parallel lines until you reach the ear.*

*4. Comb your fingers through the hair and slowly allow your partner to take the weight of the head as you change hands and repeat the whole technique over the other side of the head.*

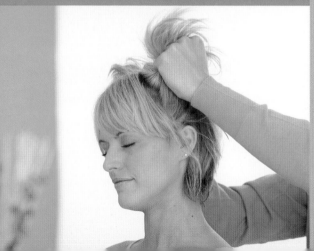

# Tapping, hacking

Light tapping produces a counterbalancing reaction within the whole head. It sends energizing ripples through the skull and brain, which wakes up all of the cells. If your head starts to feel sluggish during the day, a light, vigorous tapping on your own head can really get you going again. It can reduce the pain of headache caused by air conditioning or computer work, loosen up your neck and shoulders, and free your arms from the stiffness of immobility.

Hacking is a stronger massage technique than tapping, using the full weight of the hands and lower arms. Hacking works at a deeper level which frees up tension in the lower tissues within the muscles.

**TAPPING**
*This can be done with both hands, but if your partner is very relaxed, support the head with one hand and work with the other.*

**TWO-HAND TAPPING**
*Starting at the hairline, use all fingers of both hands to tap back to the base of the neck, across the shoulders, and down the upper arms (01). Repeat two or three times, varying the line to cover the whole head, but always sweeping across the shoulders.*

**SINGLE-HAND TAPPING**
*Support the head with one hand and use the other to tap over the other side of the head and out along the shoulder two or three times. Repeat on the other side.*

**HACKING**
*Work with both hands, rapidly bouncing your hands off the head (02). Cover the whole of the head, neck, shoulders, and down over the upper back. This should be a whipping action.*

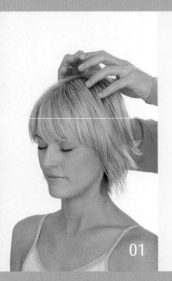

01

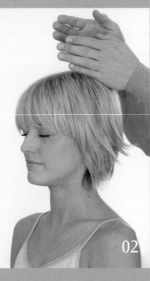

02

# Ear massage

There are over two hundred acupuncture points within the ears which acupuncturists use to reach every part of your body. These can also be stimulated by pressure to help tone, stimulate, detox, and de-stress your whole being.

**NOTES AND SUGGESTIONS**
The ears will probably feel very hot when you have finished this massage.

*1. Take hold of both of your partner's ears at the top, close to the head, between your finger and thumb.*
*2. Rub firmly while moving your grasp down around the outer edge of the ears to the lobes (01).*
*3. When you reach the lobes, pull down for a count of ten (02). Return to the tops and move down one finger width into the shells of the ears (03).*
*4. Repeat in a circular direction, following the shape of the ear. Massage firmly into all the nooks and crannies. When you have completed this, hold your hands over the ears for several moments.*

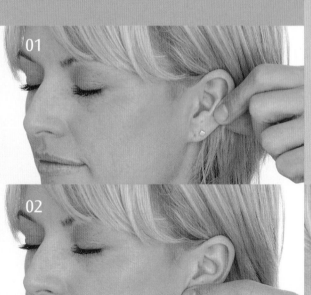

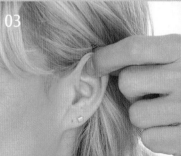

# Face stroking

This movement tones and conditions all of your facial muscles, encouraging them to fight against the forces of gravity. You will actually feel your face expanding as the tension dissolves away and wrinkles ease out.

*1. Allow your partner to rest their head against you.*
*2. With both hands meeting under the chin, lightly stroke in an upward and outward direction (see right). Move your hands to meet under the nose and stroke again. Move your hands so that they meet on the nose and, avoiding the eyes, stroke upward and outward once more. Place your hands so that they meet on the forehead and stroke upward and outward again. Repeat this three or four times.*

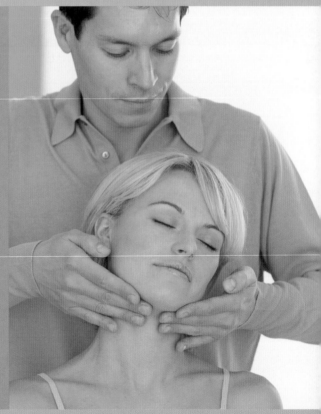

# Muscle resistance

This not only wakes up your face and head but is also very good for strengthening the facial muscles and reducing wrinkle formation. It also helps with eye strain, sinus problems, and head and facial tension.

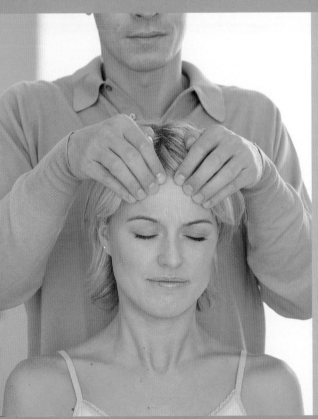

*1. Place all of the fingertips of both hands in the centre of your partner's forehead (see left). Ask them to tense the muscles under your fingertips for a count of 10, then release.*
*2. Move your fingertips two finger widths apart so that you are working toward the temples and working both sides of the face at the same time. Tense and release.*
*3. Move your fingers two finger widths again and repeat. Do this until you reach the temples. Move your fingers to meet in the middle of the nose and tense and release, even over the eyes, until you reach the ears. Move down again to cover the area from the nose to the chin, tense and release.*
*4. Hold the sides of the face for a few moments before breaking the contact.*

# CHAPTER SIX

# The whole works

The end of a day – whether it has been busy, stressful, or just plain fun, is a time when you can relax, fall into a wonderful soothing bath, and then enjoy an evening just for the two of you. An hour or so of unwinding massage provides healing, rejuvenating bliss – the power of touch at its most potent.

Techniques taken from Shiatsu, holistic massage, Tantric massage, head massage, and other gentle, soothing routines can release all the tensions and stresses at the root of many of today's health problems. These techniques do not rely on strong manipulation, but on persuasion, relaxation, and release. Every cell in the body communicates with every other and if one part of the body feels under attack, this gives rise to tension, which can transmit itself to every part of our being. However, the deep, gentle techniques of holistic therapies will make us confident that there will be no sudden surprises and so will more readily submit to releasing stress.

The fascia, a fibrous connective tissue that runs through our bodies, touching and communicating with every living part, is very sensitive to stress. In fact, prolonged stress can produce solid knots and areas of almost unbreakable tension within this fascia, triggering deep-seated illness in organs such as the heart, lungs, and intestines. The strength of the fascia can vary from a fine web to strong diaphragms. If the membrane around your joints is under prolonged tension, it can cause misalignment. Regular deep relaxation, of which massage is a major part, can do much to relieve this imbalance.

Starting with a meditation that will connect you and your partner and release the pull of the outside world, then moving on to work with the yang protector areas of the body and, finally, with the more sensitive yin areas, this routine will allow body, mind, and spirit to completely renew and refresh themselves at the deepest level.

# Creating the atmosphere

Prepare a cosy space in which to perform your massage. As the floor is the working area for this massage, ensure that you have enough room to allow your partner to lie full length in comfort, and to enable you to move freely without feeling cramped.

Place a couple of duvets or folded blankets on the floor, so that you have enough padding all around your partner to kneel or sit on. Have two or three small pillows or cushions to place under the head and shoulders when needed and a sheet or light blanket to cover your partner in the closing stages.

Play your favourite soft music to lead you through the massage unless you would prefer silence.

Use a light, subtle fragrance of your favourite oil in a carrier oil such as grapeseed on your hands, as this can help you both to move into a healing, meditative state. Oil burners are also useful, but take care with the strength of the fragrance.

If it is daylight outside draw the curtains. If you are not using oils in a burner or on your hands, then scented candles can provide aroma and soft lighting.

Good ventilation and an even, warm temperature are important. Sudden gusts of hot air from a fan heater can be distracting, even on a cool night, while a cool breeze in a hot room can be very pleasurable.

While you are setting up your room try to slow your breathing. Allow your movements to flow rhythmically. See this as a ritual for communication between you, your partner, and the universe.

Now try the meditation on pp.96–7 to synchronize your breathing and clear your energy flow.

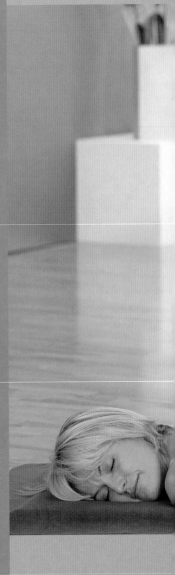

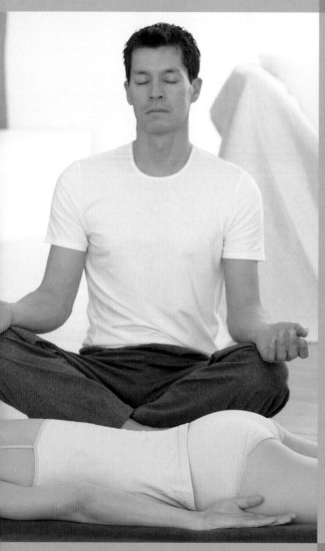

### CHOOSING YOUR OILS

*You can blend your own mixture of oils if you prefer. For a deep, woody scent you could use a few drops of frankincense with sandalwood. For a soft, floral aroma blend a few drops of geranium with chamomile. For a fresh, fruity scent use a few drops of lemongrass with basil. Lemongrass can also be used with the woody oils to lighten their scent. Frankincense can be added to the floral or citrus oils to deepen their perfume. But don't use too many oils in a mixture or they will fight each other.*

# Amber meditation

This meditation will help to clear your energies and those of the room. Amber is a fossilized plant resin. It is considered very healing and acts by absorbing negative energy and emitting positive energy. It is a calming, soothing, and relaxing stone which your partner may like to hold during the massage. Alternatively, place a few amber crystals around the room to help rebalance any negativity released during the treatment.

## NOTES AND SUGGESTIONS

Work on a well-padded floor, using a couple of duvets or folded blankets.

For the massage, have your partner lie face down, forehead supported, so that the head and neck are straight and the arms are down by the sides.

If you find that your hands are feeling heavy, buzzy, or as if they are cloaked in cotton wool, give them a hard shake.

Visualize the static leaving your hands and disappearing into the earth. This will disperse any dense energy that you may have gathered while you were working.

1. Sit a relaxed arm's length opposite your partner. Gaze into each other's eyes for a few moments to see into each other's hearts.
2. Place your dominant hand on your partner's heart, placing your free hand over their hand that is on your heart (see right). Synchronize your breathing.
3. Close your eyes and imagine a warm amber mist filling the room. Allow the mist to move over your skin, sliding like a breeze.
4. Put your awareness into this feeling, allowing it to touch every part of you.
5. Feel the mist circling and swirling around the room, allowing your awareness to be carried with it. If thoughts from the day intrude, observe and let go.
6. Feel the mist moving under your skin, slipping just under the surface, moving deeper within you.
7. Feel the mist circling between the two of you, running from your hand to your partner's heart and

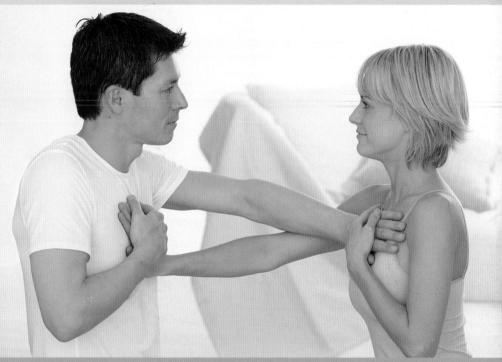

back from their hand to your
heart. Allow this mist to
circle for a few moments
to build the connection
between you.
8. Feel the circle growing
out from you into the room,
filling the room. Allow this

circle to flow for a few
moments.
9. Feel golden sparks
shooting throughout the
circle, energizing and
cleansing the whole room.
10. Now slowly allow the
mist to spiral down into the

earth, taking with it any
negativity and worries of
the day, leaving behind a
soothing, calm atmosphere.
11. Slowly have your partner
lie face down and take
position for your first
massage move.

# Tiger's claw

The full sequence of this massage moves energy at a very deep cellular level.

## NOTES AND SUGGESTIONS

Work with both hands at the same time, following the rising yang and descending yin energy flow. Stand at your partner's feet. Hold your hands in a claw shape, with strong fingers. The hands are strong, but the touch is light. Move in a continuous flow, lightly running over the whole body. If you are going to do the whole massage sequence below, end the tiger's claw at the head, before turning your partner over.

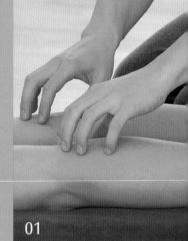

01

1. Start at the ankles and lightly stroke up the back of the calves to the knees (01). Move your hands out to the sides of the legs and stroke back down to the feet . Repeat three times, ending on the rising stroke, just behind the knees.
2. Continue the upward stroke over the buttocks to the hips (02). Move to the outside and downstroke to the knees. Repeat this line three times, ending on the upstroke level with the hips.
3. Continue the upstroke to the shoulders (03). Move your hands out to the arms and stroke down the inner arms to the hands. Stroke up the outside of the arms and down the inside of the arms three times, ending on an upstroke at the shoulders.
4. Stroke both hands down your partner's sides to the hips. Move in toward the spine and stroke upward toward their shoulders (this follows the governing vessel). Repeat this three times, ending at the neck.
5. For the neck and head you will need to close up the claw to the thumb and two or three fingers. Lightly stroke up the centre back of the neck to the crown of the head. Move your fingers out to each side of the head and stroke down to the base of the neck. Repeat three times.
6. If you are not going on to do the complete tiger's claw sequence, end here and go on to cat walking on back (see p.100). Otherwise, turn your partner over and continue.
7. Starting at the head,

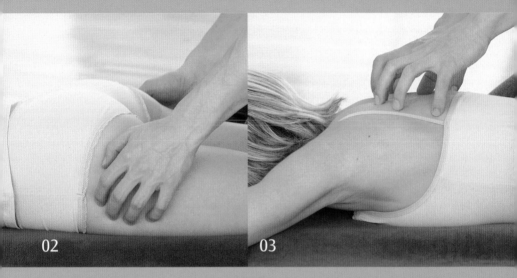

02

03

lightly stroke down the centre of the face and throat. At the base of the neck move your hands out to the sides and upstroke across the ears to the top of the head. Repeat three times, ending at the top of the sternum on a downstroke.

8. Move out to the arms and continue the downstroke over the outer sides of the arms, ending at the hands. Stroke up the inner arms to the shoulders. Repeat this three times, ending on an upstroke at the shoulders.

9. Move your hands back to the sternum. With one hand following the other down the centre of the body (this follows the conceptual vessel), move down until you reach the hara (lower abdomen). At the tanden, which is two finger widths below the navel, move your hands out to your partner's sides and stroke upward. Repeat three times, ending on a sideways stroke, stopping level with the tops of the thighs.

10. Stroke down the front of the legs to the knees. Move to the outer side of the legs and stroke upward to the top of the legs. Repeat three times, ending on a downstroke at the knees.

11. Continue the downstroke to the feet. Do not work the soles as the light touch will tickle, destroying the relaxing effect. Move to the sides of the ankles and stroke up the sides of the legs to the knees. Repeat three times. End at the feet, holding them for a few moments.

# Cat walking on back

This is a very deep treatment which works right down into the build-up of tight muscles that may not have fully relaxed for many years. You will feel a lot younger after only a few minutes of cat walking. Your stance will be more fluid and mobile and you will walk and move in a lighter way. This is a wonderful stretch for an aching lower back.

**CAUTION**
■ *Care must be taken in cases of clinical back problems or conditions.*

*1. Position yourself above and facing your partner's head. Place your hands on the back, just below the neck and about two finger widths either side of the spine (01). Angle your fingers 45 degrees from the spine.*
*2. Kneel on one knee to improve your reach and balance. Slow your breathing to match your partner's, as* this will connect the two of you. Try to hold a feeling of warmth moving between the two of you throughout the whole treatment. Move slowly and try to feel your partner's response.
*3. Walk hand over hand down the back, being careful not to put any weight on the spine (02). When you reach the base of the spinal area* hold that position for a moment (03). You should let your whole body weight rest on your hands.
*4. Now slowly push yourself back, hand over hand, to your original position. Repeat at least three times.*

01

02

03

# Side stretch

This technique is excellent for loosening up the entire back, releasing tension and pain.

## NOTES AND SUGGESTIONS
If your partner has a very long back you may need to move two palm widths down after step 2 to reach the final stretch.

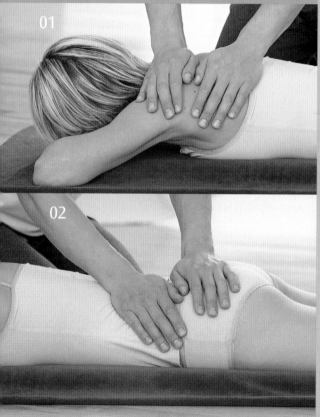

*1. Move to your partner's right side. Starting on the shoulder area, place the heels of both hands about two finger widths away from the left side of the spine, with your fingers at right angles to the spine (01). Lean your weight slowly on to your hands and develop a push that will move the muscles of the upper back to stretch away from the spine. Hold for a count of ten.*
*2. Release and move your hands about two palm widths down the back. Put the heels of your hands about two finger widths away from the left side of the spine, fingers at right angles to the spine, and lean into the stretch, dropping your weight slowly on to your hands. Hold for a count of ten, then release.*
*3. Repeat, moving another two palm widths down the body. You should have one hand on the left hip, one on the waist (02). Angle the stretch at about 60 degrees to the spine, pushing out and down.*
*4. Move to the opposite side and repeat the sequence.*

# Cross stretching

This stretches all the muscles of the back in directions that move the muscle fibres over each other, helping to release toxin build-up within the muscles. It encourages a good flow of blood to all of your back muscles and frees up any locks in your spinal area.

**CAUTION**
Great care must be taken if your partner has clinical back problems.

1. Place your right hand on the right hip and your left hand on the left shoulder blade. Slowly drop your weight on to your hands in a crossways stretch. Hold for a count of three (01).
2. Release and change your hand positions so that your right hand is on the left hip and your left hand is on the right shoulder blade. Drop into the stretch and hold for a count of three (02).
3. Release. Leaving your right hand on the left hip, place your left hand under the right rib cage. Drop your weight into the stretch. Hold for a count of three (03).
4. Release, move your right hand over to the right hip and cross your left hand over to hold the left rib cage. Drop into the stretch. Hold for a count of three (04).
5. Release. Now cross your arms level with your partner's waist, placing your hands on their body, pointing away from each other, and pushing away from the spine in each case. Stretch, hold for a count of three (05), and release.

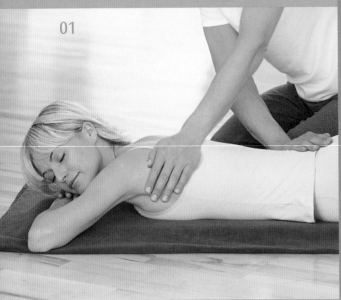

01

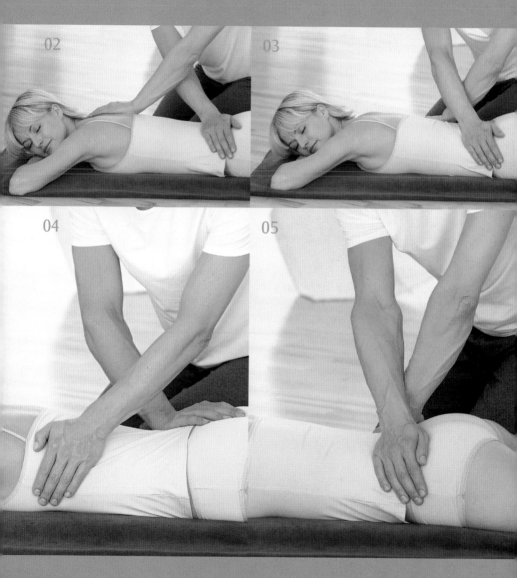

# Back massage techniques

## HACKING

You and your partner should breathe deeply during this movement to maximize the oxygenation of your bodies. Hold your hands loosely so that your fingers curl naturally. With swift, free-flowing wrists and hands, hack lightly over the whole back – this should be a whipping rather than a beating motion. It should be done with care, since, if performed too vigorously by untrained hands, it could hurt your wrists. Starting from one buttock move in a circular direction up the back, across the shoulders, down the other side of the back, and over the buttocks. Continue this movement for three to four circuits. Then rest. This is very energizing and enlivening for both of you (see also p.88).

## BACK ROTATIONS

Hold your partner's shoulder with one hand, referred to as the listening hand. You don't need to pay too much attention to this hand, just be aware of any changes in your partner as you work with your other hand. With the fingers of your working hand, start about two finger widths away from the spine, at shoulder level, and move away from the spine and your listening hand. The pressure should be firm without being painful. Work your fingers in small rotations over a small area for a count of three to five (01, 02). Then move about three finger widths in the direction of your partner's side and repeat. Continue until you reach your partner's side, then come back to the spine. Drop your hand about a palm

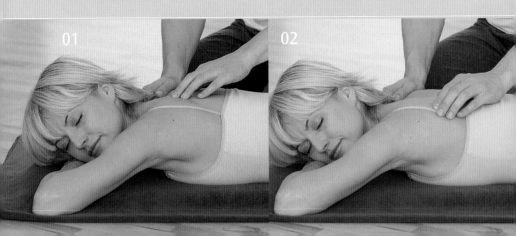

01

02

width down the back and start the rotations again. Cover that side of the back then move to the other side of the body, changing hands so that the listening hand and the working hand swap places, and cover the rest of the back with rotations. If the pressure is kept firm, this technique gives a deep soothing massage that will break down any long-held tension.

### WORKING THE VERTEBRAE
Still holding your partner's shoulder with the listening hand, loosen the spine by working each vertebra. Use your thumb and three fingers of your working hand to grasp each vertebra in turn and move it in a circular motion for a count of three (03), starting at the base of the neck and working down to the coccyx. This frees up the whole spine, making it mobile and supple.

### TIGER'S CLAW
This is a short, figure-of-eight variation, for the back only. You can use one hand or both. If you are working with one hand, use your other to "listen". Start at the middle top of the back, holding your hand lightly in the shape of a claw, with strong fingers. Stroke in a figure of eight across your partner's upper back for seven circuits. Then, slide your hand down to mid back, without breaking the rhythm, and do another seven circuits (04). Move down again to the lower back and repeat the seven circuits.

If you want to work with both hands you will find details of the technique on pp.98–9.

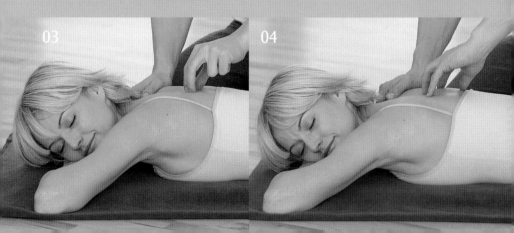

# Palming down legs

This is a light massage which will encourage good
circulation of blood and lymph fluids within your legs.
It relaxes the large muscles in your legs, helping to
ease out back and leg pains caused by bad posture.
Massaging can be just as beneficial for the giver.
If you allow yourself to move freely and work to
your extreme, your balance and flexibility
will improve greatly.

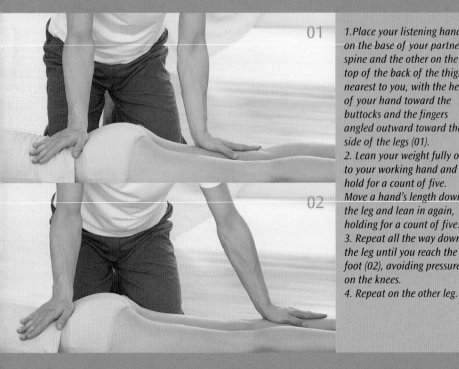

01

02

1. Place your listening hand
on the base of your partner's
spine and the other on the
top of the back of the thigh
nearest to you, with the heel
of your hand toward the
buttocks and the fingers
angled outward toward the
side of the legs (01).
2. Lean your weight fully on
to your working hand and
hold for a count of five.
Move a hand's length down
the leg and lean in again,
holding for a count of five.
3. Repeat all the way down
the leg until you reach the
foot (02), avoiding pressure
on the knees.
4. Repeat on the other leg.

# Wringing out calves

This is a more vigorous massage which works strongly on the muscles of the calves. The movement is like that used when wringing out wet clothes, and it literally squeezes toxins out of the muscle fibres. It also works to dispel any stagnant blood that has pooled in the lower legs.

**CAUTION**
■ *This massage should not be attempted if your partner has varicose veins.*

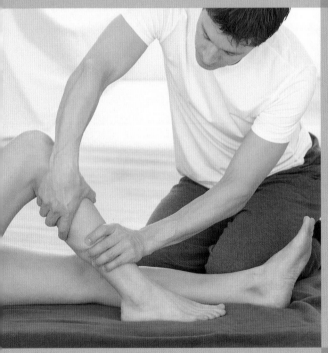

*1. Hold one of your partner's calves with two hands and, starting just below the knee, wring out as you would a wet garment, moving down the leg to the foot (see left).*
*2. Repeat on the other leg.*
*3. End by sitting at your partner's feet and holding them for a few moments. Pick up the feet and support both of them over your lap. Now begin working the feet and ankles (see pp.108–9).*

# Rotating ankles

The load-bearing joints of your ankles take a huge amount of strain on even the most sedentary day. Imagine holding your own weight in your hands as you get out of bed in the morning. It would be quite an effort, yet that is the strain your ankles take every time you get up from a chair, climb stairs, or do anything that moves your weight from one foot to the other. To combat this strain, your ankle joint can, over time, sometimes hold a permanent tension. This can cause pain and stiffness and also trap waste cellular matter within the joint. Rotating your ankles in a way that is not load-bearing can help to free this stiffness, improving the overall mobility and strength of your ankle joints.

*CAUTION*
■ *Care must be taken if your partner has any damage to the joints.*

1. *Hold one of your partner's ankles in one hand (01). Grasp the foot with the other hand and move it in a smooth circular rotation (02). Be careful not to cause any pain, but try to explore the full movement of the ankle. Work first in one direction, then the other.*
2. *Continue with the stretching (see p.109) and a massage (see p.110) before moving on to the other foot.*

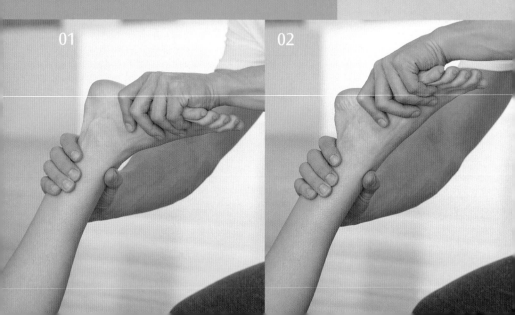

01

02

# Stretching feet

As your ankle starts to stiffen, more strain is placed on other areas of your feet. This sequence will ease out any tense muscles and stretch the tendons of your ankle and foot. It will also free up any immobility in your toes, helping your balance and bringing a lighter, flowing quality to your gait. You'll walk taller and feel more energetic after this massage.

*1. Hold your partner's ankle with one hand. Place the working hand over the heel and, lean into your hand with your forearm. Press it along the sole of the foot, stretching it as far as it will go, with the toes moving toward the knee (see left).*
*2. Change the position of your working hand and hold the top of the foot.*
*3. Now stretch the foot in the other direction, pointing the toes as far as they will go.*
*4. Finish this foot with rotations and toe pulling (see p.110) before repeating the whole sequence on the other foot.*

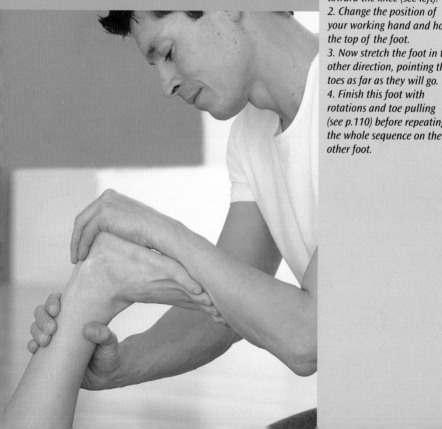

# Rotations over the feet and toe pulling

This increases the flexibility of the feet and helps to move any toxin build-up. It also works many of the meridians of the body, such as the lung, large intestine, stomach, spleen, heart, small intestine, bladder, kidney, liver, and gall bladder, promoting overall good health and well-being.

## NOTES AND SUGGESTIONS
This is a simple massage which you can also use as a self-treatment to relieve tired feet and help you get through the most trying day. As the old saying goes – "What goes on in your feet shows in your face."

1. *Support your partner's foot by holding the top of the foot, with the sole facing you.*
2. *Starting at the heel and moving along the outer edge of the foot work your thumb quite firmly (light pressure tickles) in small circles for a count of five in each position (01). Move down the edge about two finger widths and repeat until you reach the little toe.*
3. *Grasp the little toe firmly and pull, holding the stretch for a count of three.*
4. *Go back to the heel, move one finger width in toward the inner side of the foot, and repeat the sequence.*
5. *Do this three more times until you have covered the whole foot and pulled each toe in turn (02).*
6. *Now repeat, this time doing the rotations with your fingers over the top of the foot and following four lines between the bones of the foot down toward the toes. Repeat the whole sequence from the ankle rotation (p.108) on the other foot.*

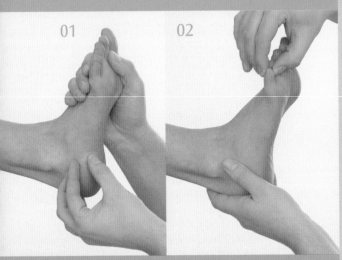

01

02

# Finishing off

This closing sequence follows the rising yang and descending yin energies of the body, which helps to smooth out any remaining ripples of unbalanced energy in the back. It also pulls your energy away from your partner as they turn over for the front massage.

## NOTES AND SUGGESTIONS

If your partner is very relaxed at this point and is close to sleep, closing the back with an energy sweep means that you can leave the massage here without your partner feeling only half done.

*1. Using your whole hand, stroke up the back of the calves to the knees and down the sides of the legs to the feet three times (01).*
*2. On the third sweep continue up the back of the legs to the hips and then down to the knees three times (02).*
*3. Sweep up the back to the shoulders and down the sides to the base of the spine three times (03).*
*4. Ask your partner to turn over and continue.*

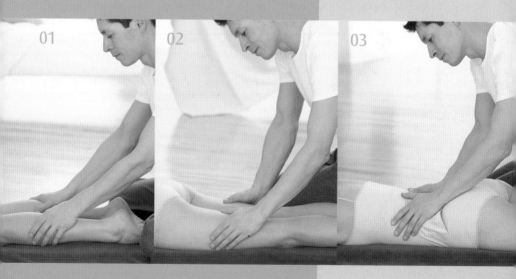

# Knee swings

This is a lovely stretch for the lower spine. It gently moves apart the vertebrae of the mid and lower spine, releasing any long-held tension.

## NOTES AND SUGGESTIONS
If your partner can't relax into the swing or feels insecure about you being able to carry their weight, you can simply lean back while holding their knees and stretch the spine without lifting the body from the floor. This way you will both gain confidence in each other's abilities and eventually you and your partner will be able to relax fully into this exercise.

**CAUTION**
■ *Great care must be taken if your partner has a clinical back problem.*

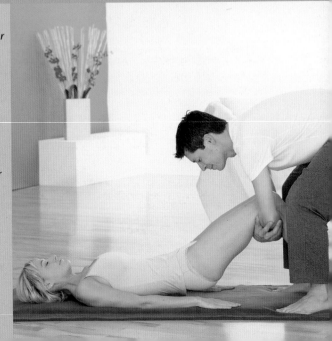

1. Stand with your legs apart, feet either side of your partner's knees. Pick up her knees (see right). If the legs remain tense, ask her to relax and allow her feet to drop to the floor.
2. Use your bent knees to support your elbows. Lean back to lift your partner's lower body off the floor.
3. Gently swing your partner from side to side about six to eight times.

# Knee stretches

This is a more strenuous stretch, which works deeply into the rotating action of the back. Your partner will feel wonderful after it.

## NOTES AND SUGGESTIONS

You may find that your partner will resist this stretch as it is moving the body in an unusual way. If you feel them tensing ask them to make a deep inhalation and exhalation. You should be able to stretch a further 3–4 cm (1–1½ in) more and this will release their back. You may even find that their back crackles slightly as it frees up. But don't go so far as to cause pain.

*1. Push your partner's knees up toward her chest, and hold for a count of five (01). To extend the stretch, lower the knees to the floor on one side (02), but do not allow her opposite shoulder to lift. If that happens, use one hand to hold down the knees and the other to hold down the shoulder. Hold for five.*
*2. Raise the knees to the centre and stretch to the other side.*
*3. Come back to centre. Slide your hands to grasp the ankles, shake them to loosen the whole body, and slowly lower the legs to the floor.*

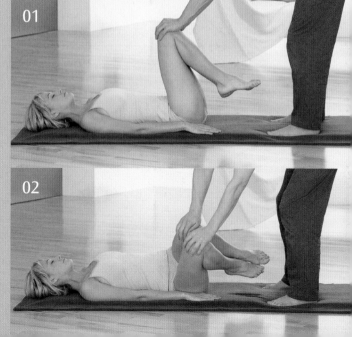

01

02

# Arm stretching/wringing

Arm stretching uses the weight of your partner's body to gently release tension in their arms, shoulders, and upper back. By stretching the arms in this way you are assisting the flow of blood within the fibres of the muscles and easing those fibres over each other, allowing toxins and cellular debris to be dissolved by the blood and lymph fluids and carried away. The muscles themselves are also being stretched and released like an elastic band, which helps to relax the whole of the upper body.

**ARM STRETCHING**

*1. Stand behind your partner's head and take her hands.*

*2. Holding the wrists in both of your hands bend your knees and use them to support your elbows as you lean back and stretch your partner's upper spine (see p.112). Don't lift the body from the floor as the neck could twist uncomfortably. Just put their arms under tension and shake gently.*

*3. If you wish, from this position you could sit down on the floor, place your feet on your partner's shoulders, and stretch the arms by pulling with your hands and pushing with your feet. Don't push too hard, just enough to ease out any shoulder stiffness. Return your partner's arms to their sides.*

**ARM WRINGING**

*1. Sit by your partner's side and hold the opposite upper arm with both hands.*

*2. Work your way down the arm using a wringing motion (see left). Massage the hand, then work on the other arm.*

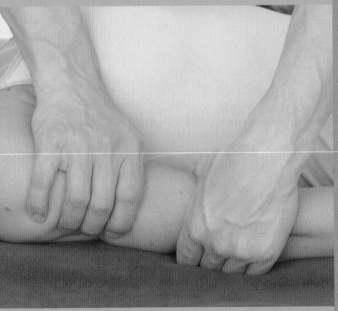

# Hand squeezing

This is a more intensive treatment for the hands, which works more strongly on the tissues to move any deep build-up of cellular debris and toxin deposits. This helps to free off any long-term stiffness in the muscles and joints, particularly in the hands and wrists. You will also cover many of the meridians that are found in the feet, giving a well-balanced treatment which will help to maintain good health. The squeezing can also be used as quick, effective, refreshing, and pain-relieving self-treatment.

*1. Massage your partner's hand by squeezing it between your fingers and thumb as if making pastry, rubbing with your fingers on the back of the hand and with your thumbs over the palm (see left).*
*2. Work strongly from the heel of the hand to the fingertips, starting at the outer edge, up the little finger, and progressing over the hand toward the thumb.*
*3. Repeat the sequence of arm wringing and squeezing on the other hand.*

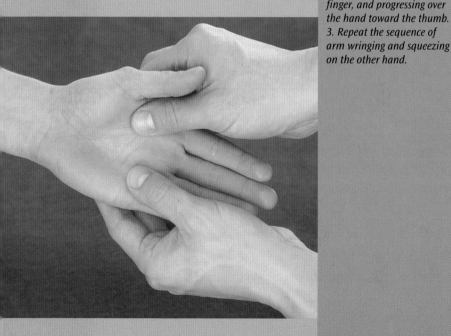

# Abdomen: palm rolls

This is a particularly good treatment for anyone with digestive or elimination problems, as the palm rolls stimulate the organs within your abdominal area. Working from right to left encourages the flow of waste products through the intestines, the circulation of blood and other fluids through the kidneys and liver, and a healthy bowel action. Health problems such as irritable bowel syndrome (IBS) and Crohn's disease can be helped by the calming effect of palm rolls and the bowl (see p.117). Palm rolls also gently stimulate the meridians that pass through the abdominal area.

## NOTES AND SUGGESTIONS
Releasing emotional problems can trigger a reaction that may last for a few days, but your partner will feel very much better and freer for this release.

*1. Sit at your partner's right side, level with the abdomen. Place your hands on the abdomen, fingers closed (01). Hold for a moment to allow your partner to relax fully.*
*2. Lean your weight gently on to the heels of your hands (02). In a wavelike motion slowly roll your weight through your hands to the fingertips (03).*
*3. Lean back to return your weight to the starting position and repeat the wave seven to ten times. The rolling action should be smooth and flowing with medium pressure.*

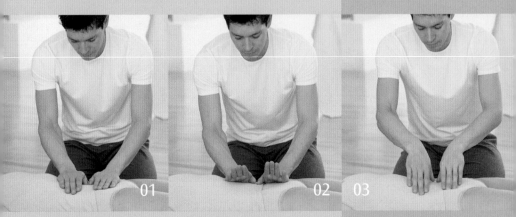

01  02  03

# Abdomen: bowl

The bowl is very good for digestive and elimination problems. It is a gentler action than palm rolls and is very soothing and calming. It also stimulates the yin meridians which run from the head down through the body and into the feet. This gives a gentle workout for the conceptual/directing vessel, stomach, kidney, lung (through the lung extension), spleen, liver, and large intestine channels. It can help to stretch the fascia within the abdominal area. It is very calming and, as it also works the solar plexus and hara (lower abdomen) areas, it can help to release emotional problems.

## NOTES AND SUGGESTIONS
As for palm rolls (see p.116).

*1. In the same position as for the palm rolls, lift the inner sides of your hands so that they form a bowl shape (01).*
*2. Rock your weight in a circular motion so that it rolls clockwise around the rim of the bowl. Move with your whole body for seven to ten circuits.*
*3. When you have completed this, lightly hold your hands over the abdomen (02). Hold this position for a few moments. Observe your partner's breathing, slowly allowing their body to fall away from your hands.*
*4. Cover your partner with a sheet or light blanket and seat yourself at their head for the neck and shoulder workout and head massage.*

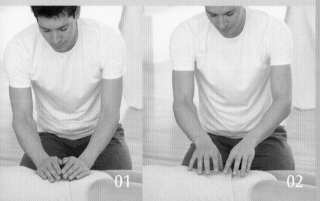

01        02

# Neck and shoulder workout

Strong massage around your neck and shoulders releases tension headaches, eye strain, facial pain, and stiff muscles in your neck, shoulders, arms, and hands.

*1. Sit behind your partner, place your hands above her shoulders (01), and slide them under the shoulders, close to the spine.*

*2. Using your partner's body weight to increase the strength of the work, make claws and, moving one hand after the other in an upward rolling action, work into the shoulder area and neck for a slow count of ten (02).*

*3. Place the inside edges of your hands under the base of your partner's neck, with your forefingers touching the neck and your little fingers against the floor.*

*4. Working hand over hand, pull strongly upward under your partner's neck, from base to top. Repeat this action for a slow count of ten, ending with one hand supporting the base of your partner's skull.*

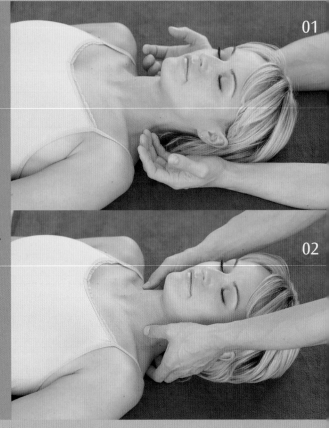

# Head rotations, combing, stroking, pressure, hair pulling

These techniques are helpful for stress and headaches.

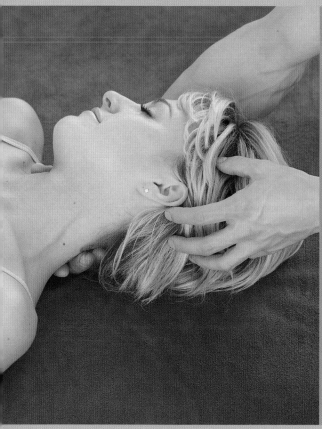

### ROTATIONS

*1. Tilt your partner's head to one side (see left). With the fingers of your free hand, starting at the base of your partner's skull, rotate upward toward the crown. The pressure should be firm without pulling or causing any pain.*

*2. When you reach the crown, move the head to face forward. Still supporting the head with one hand, continue the rotations right up to the hairline.*

*3. Using both hands, one each side of the head, and starting as far back as you can reach, work the rotations along the sides of the head until you reach the hairline.*

### COMBING AND STROKING

*Comb your fingers upward and outward through the hair and stroke gently down over the hair. Repeat as many times as you wish.*

### PRESSURE

*1. Support your partner's head with one hand and turn it to one side. With the fingers of the other hand, start at the base of the skull and exert a firm pressure for a count of three (01).*

*2. Move two finger widths up toward the crown and press in with your fingers for a count of three. Repeat until you reach the crown.*

*3. Turn the head to the front and continue with both hands along the sides of the head to the hairline, just in front of the ears.*

*4. Press both thumbs across the forehead, from the sides toward the centre (02).*

*5. When your thumbs meet, change direction. Work from the centre of the forehead to the crown (03). Bring your thumbs to the forehead and out two finger widths.*

*6. Work two lines parallel to the centre, toward the crown. Repeat two finger widths out again, to the outer edge of the head, before it curves down. Go over the whole head with more combing and stroking.*

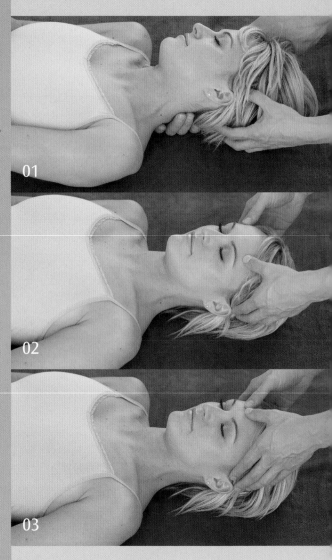

## HAIR PULLING

1. Slide both of your hands, with open fingers, through the hair at the side of your partner's head until you have collected a good handful of hair.

2. Close up your fingers and pull outward in a direction perpendicular to the scalp (01). Repeat all over the head. This is a wonderful technique for relieving a headache.

3. Go over the whole head with combing and stroking (02). You can also follow this with any of the techniques you choose from the full head massage sequence (see pp.78–91).

4. Close the treatment by holding your partner's head for a few moments before slowly withdrawing your hands (03).

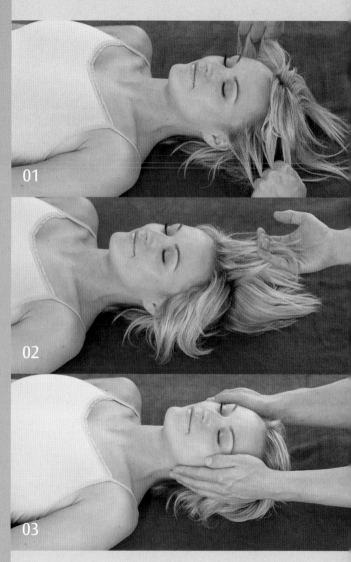

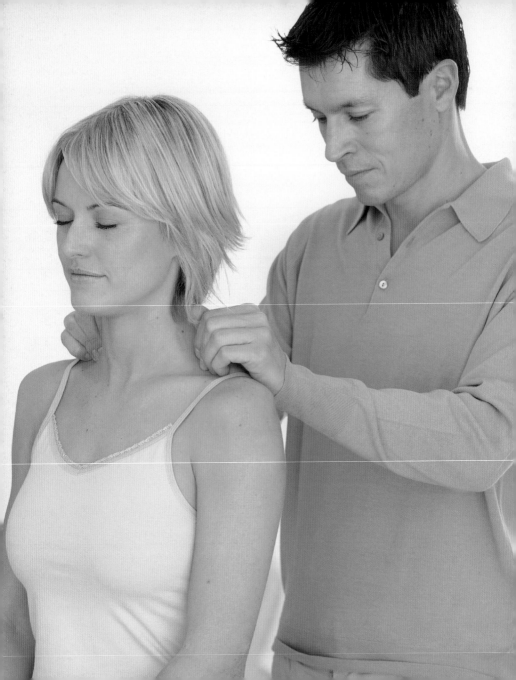

# Further reading

Alexander, Jane
*Five-Minute Healer*
Gaia Books, 1999

Baker, Ian A.
*The Tibetan Art of Healing*
Thames and Hudson, 1997

Bentley, Eilean
*Step-by-Step Head Massage*
Gaia Books, 2000

Burmeister, Alice and
Monte, Tom
*The Touch of Healing
(Jin Shin Jyutsu)*
Bantam Books, 1997

Chaitow, Leon
*Positional Release
Techniques*
Churchill Livingstone, 1996

Chia, Mantak
*Awaken Healing Energy
Through the Tao*
Aurora Press,1983

Evans, Mark
*Instant Stretches*
Lorenz Books, 1996

Frantzis, B.K.
*Opening the Energy Gates
of Your Body*
North Atlantic Books, 1993

Gach, Michael Reed
*Acupressure*
Piatkus, 1990

Gillanders, Ann
*BPG Reflexology*
Gaia Books, 2002

Jarmey, Chris and
Mojay, Gabriel
*Shiatsu – The Complete
Guide*
Thorsons, 1991

Jarmey, Chris and
Tindall, John
*Acupressure for Common
Ailments*
Gaia Books, 1991

Lundberg, Paul
*The Book of Shiatsu*
Gaia Books, 1992

Masunaga, Shizut and
Ohashi, Wataru
*Zen Shiatsu*
Japan Publications, 1977

Melody
*Love is in the Earth*
Earth-Love Pub, 1995

Metzger, Wolfgang and
Zhou, Peifang
*Tai Chi Chuan and Qigong*
Sterling books, 1996

Rich, Penny
*Practical Aromatherapy*
Siena Books, 1996

Shen, Peijian
*Massage for Pain Relief*
Gaia Books, 1996

Szwillus, Marlisa
*Mood Food*
Gaia Books, 1999

Taylor, Kylea
*The Breathwork Experience*
Hanford Mead, 1994

# Index

## A

abdomen
  bowl 117
  massage 58
  pain 41, 72
  palm rolls 116
  problems 65
acupressure 6, 15, 16
acupuncture 15, 89, 122
ailments 40–3
alternate nostril breathing 51
amber meditation 94, 96–7
ankle rotation 108
anxiety 16, 19, 40, 50
arm
  massage 57
  pinch 82
  squeeze 115
  stretch 114
  swing 74–5
aromatherapy 6, 15, 20–3
arthritis 9
asthma 11, 19
atmosphere 94–5

## B

back
  cat walking 100
  clinical problems 102, 112
  massage 58, 81, 104–5
  rotations 104
backache 16, 40, 78, 100, 106
bath massage 37
bone disease 86
bowl 116, 117
breathing 30, 34–5, 50, 53, 61
  alternate nostril 51
  deep 69
  difficulties 16, 19, 40–1, 61
  exercises 50
  synchronizing 94
bronchitis 19
buses 48, 49

## C

calves 107
cancer 86
candles 94
carrier oils 21, 94
cat walking 100
cerebrospinal fluid 80
chakra meditation 7, 44–7
circular breath 34
coffee break massage 64–7
colds 16, 19, 41, 84
colour visualization 62–3
combing 86, 119
concentration 7, 16, 76–7, 80
connective tissue 93
constipation 9, 41, 58, 65
cramp 19, 30, 49
Crohn's disease 11, 116
cross stretches 102
crystals 6–7, 11, 24–7, 76, 96, 122

## D

daydreaming 11
deep vein thrombosis (DVT) 59
depression 11, 16, 19, 86
detoxing 89
diarrhoea 58, 65
driving 48, 49, 83

## E

ear massage 89
eczema 37
elbow rotation 83
elimination problems 116–17
emotional problems 9, 11, 19, 68, 116–17
epilepsy 21
essential oils 11, 15, 21, 36–7, 94-5
exercise 7, 52
eye strain 19, 76–7, 84, 91, 118

## F

face stroking 90
fascia 93
finishing off 111
first aid 16
flatulence 65
foot
  massage 59
  rotation 110

stretch 109
swollen 16, 78
friction rub 23
frozen shoulder 16, 68

# G

grief 19

# H

hacking 13, 23, 88, 104
hair
    pulling 85, 119, 121
    stroking 86, 119
hand massage 57
hangovers 41
head
    clearing 65, 76–7, 85
    massage 6, 11, 14, 54,
        78–91, 93
    rotation 119
    scratching 85
    shake 87
    stroking 119
headaches 7, 11, 16, 19, 41
    full body 118
    massage 84, 88
    travel 53–4
    work 64, 68, 76–7
heart disease 41
heel of hand rotations 81
high blood pressure 41
holistic massage 9, 80, 93
hyperventilation 34

# I

immune system 16, 19
Indian head massage 80
indigestion 11, 19, 41, 65,
    72–3
insomnia 11, 16, 41, 86, 119
irritable bowel syndrome
    (IBS) 11, 116

# K

kneading 12–13, 23
knee
    stretch 113
    swing 112

# L

labour pains 16
leg
    massage 59
    palming 106
lifestyle 16

# M

Masunaga, Shizuto 8
meditation 6, 11, 29, 40, 44-7
    full body 93–4, 96–7
    travel 53
    work 62–3, 74
meridians 14–15, 64, 87, 110,
    115–17
migraine 84

mineral soaks 37
muscle resistance 91
music 48, 94

# N

nausea 19, 58
neck
    loosening 68–71
    massage 55, 118
    stiff 41, 68, 78, 118
    workout 84
nosebleeds 16, 19

# O

oats 37
observation powers 29
oil burners 94
oxygen 34, 39–40, 50, 53–4,
    69, 76, 104

# P

palm rolls 116
palming 79, 106
panic attacks 40, 50
pinching 13
pregnancy 16, 21, 56
pressure 13, 15, 85, 87, 89
    full body 119, 120
    imbalances 85
    massage 54
    points 14–19, 40–3, 56,
        61, 80, 84
problem-solving 80

psoriasis 37
pummelling 13, 23

# R

raking 22
rheumatism 9, 16
rotation 12, 23, 81, 83, 85–6
    ankle 108
    back 104
    foot 110
    head 119
rush hour 11, 61, 62

# S

scalp problems 85–7
sciatica 9
self-treatment 7, 84–7, 89,
    110, 115
sensitive skin 37
shaking 39
Shiatsu 6, 8, 14–15, 44, 80,
    87, 93, 122
shoulder
    frozen 16, 68
    massage 56, 118
    pinch 82
shower massage 29, 36
side stretch 101
single-hand tapping 88
sinus problems 19, 41, 51, 54,
    91
smells 58
sore throat 16, 19

squeezing 115
stiff neck 41, 68, 78, 118
still points 84
stomach problems 41, 58
stress 11, 16, 49–50
    ear massage 89
    full body 92–3, 119
    head massage 86
    work 61, 65, 68
stretching 29, 30–1, 36, 68–71
    arm 114
    cross 102
    feet 109
    knee 113
stroking 12, 22, 29–31, 86, 90,
    119
sweeping 38, 61
swollen feet 16, 78

# T

Tantra
    breathing 34–5
    massage 93
Tao Yinn 32–3
tapping 13, 32–3, 88
techniques 12–13
temperature 36, 94
tension 11, 14, 16, 58, 61
    full body 93, 101, 108
    head massage 84, 86,
    90-1
    headaches 16, 64, 118
therapeutic massage 6, 15
tiger's claw 98–9, 105
tinnitus 84
tiredness 7, 11, 16

toe pulling 110
toning 89
toothache 19
touch 7, 8, 20, 92–3, 98
trains 11, 48, 49
travelling 7, 49–50, 54–9
tsubos 14
two-hand tapping 88

# V

varicose veins 59, 107
ventilation 94
vertebrae 105, 112
violet breath 34
visualization 11, 24–5, 40,
    61–2, 96

# W

wake-up routine 30–1
walking 49, 52–3, 76
water retention 16
wind 19
work 7, 52–3, 60–77
wringing 13
    arm 114
    calf 107
wrinkles 90
wrist pain 19

# Y

yin-yang 27, 93, 98, 117

# Acknowledgements

## Author's acknowledgements

I would like to express my grateful thanks to all my relatives, friends, students, and teachers who have helped me in many ways to complete this book, in particular, Shiatsu Master Tutor Howard Malpas, who first introduced me to complementary therapies many years ago and has since, with his wife Elsa, been a great friend and teacher. I would also like to thank all at Gaia Books, Bridgewater Books, Mike Hemsley, and models Nikki and Adam, for all their help and hard work in producing this book.

## Author details

Eilean Bentley is a member of the International Shiatsu Commission and E.A.R. (Acupuncture register). She is a master in Reiki, Seichim, and Karuna healing, and has studied Indian head massage and shamanic healing. She teaches privately and in adult and further education centres in and around London, and treats private clients as well as patients in the detox unit of an NHS hospital in the South of England. She is the author of *Step-by-Step Head Massage,* also published by Gaia Books.

## Contraindications

Massage is a very safe therapy. However, sometimes you may have some reactions which can last for a few days. These are mainly of a detoxing nature, such as headaches and digestive or emotional upsets or problems.

## Other cautions

Care is needed when treating the very young, the elderly, and those suffering from bone problems, epilepsy, clinical depression, cancer, low or high blood pressure, or who are pregnant. In these cases use only a very short, light massage.

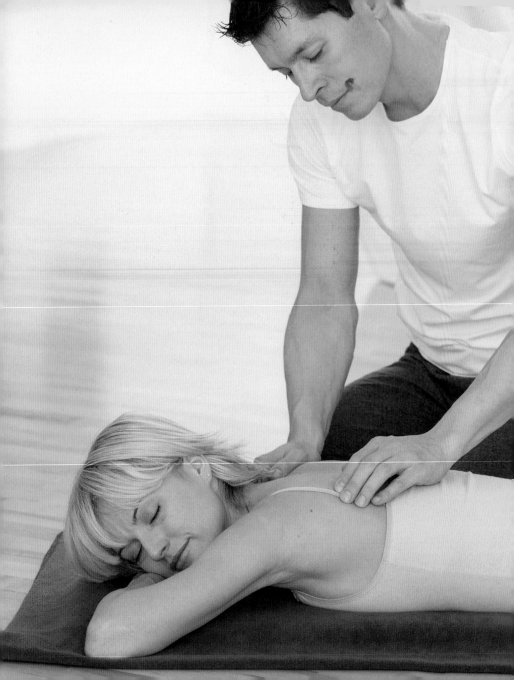

SELF

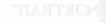

# SHEILA YEGER

# SELF PORTRAIT

AMBER LANE PRESS

All rights whatsoever in this play are strictly reserved
and application for performance, etc. must be made
before rehearsals begin to:

Cecily Ware Literary Agents
19c John Spencer Square
Canonbury, London N1 2LZ

No performance may be given unless a licence has been
obtained.

First published in 1990 by
Amber Lane Press Ltd
Cheorl House
Church Street
Charlbury, Oxon OX7 3PR

Telephone: 0608 810024

Printed in Great Britain by
Bocardo Press Ltd., Didcot, Oxfordshire

# INTRODUCTION

I first saw Gwen John's work at an exhibition held at the Anthony d'Offay Gallery in London in 1982. With no more than an amateur's interest in art, I wandered from room to room, not knowing what I was looking at or, indeed, for. Yet the paintings, small, often muted in tone, apparently so unobtrusive, spoke to me with such a distinctive and powerful voice that I immediately felt impelled to discover more about the woman who had painted them.

Soon afterwards, in conversation with Annie Castledine, I learnt that she too had become fascinated by Gwen John and by the extraordinary intensity of her portraits. It was the beginning of what was to prove a long and often difficult journey.

My search for Gwen John took me to Tenby and Haverfordwest, to the Tate Gallery and the New Forest, to Paris and Meudon, to Cardiff, Manchester and Aberystwyth. In the process I learnt a great deal about being an artist and even more about being an artist who is also a woman.

At Victoria House in Tenby, now a private hotel, the door was opened by a young mother carrying a baby. "Gwen John?" she asked wearily. She showed me to the attic room where, she believed, Gwen had slept as a child. Someone, she said, was supposed to be making a blue plaque for the front door but there was no sign of it yet. Upstairs, I stood on tiptoe to look out of the narrow window. There was no view of the sea.

At the Barbican exhibition in London I eavesdropped on the reaction of those who found the paintings "too small", "too pale", "rather insignificant", "not as good as Augustus". Some obviously preferred to watch the video and listen to the taped commentary on what seemed a shadowy life. But, for me, the 'Self Portrait', determined, steely, with its sense of contained passion, spoke volumes.

Later that year I travelled by bus to Fordingbridge in the New Forest. My son, Sam, then aged six, took a photograph of Yew Tree Cottage. Gwen John had purchased the house at Augustus's instigation but she seldom lived there. France, with its promise of seclusion and virtual anonymity, drew her back.

At the Musée Rodin in Paris I sat with Jan Shannon who had come to help translate the 3,000 love letters that Gwen wrote to the great man. While the snow fell heavily on Rodin's massive sculptures outside, we pondered on Gwen's schoolgirl French, not knowing whether to laugh or cry at her pathetic but all too familiar obsession.

The day I visited Meudon was, by an uncanny coincidence, the day that 8, rue Babie came up for auction. I climbed a wall to gaze at the wooden shack where Gwen had spent her last years as a recluse. She spent her time painting, caring for her cats, and attending the Catholic church.

Just around the corner I found the rather more substantial establishment of the philosopher Jacques Maritain and his sister-in-law Vera Oumançoff. Gwen, whose passion for this respectable lady was deemed unsuitable, was permitted to visit on Mondays only.

Up the hill stood the four-square building where Auguste Rodin had lived and worked and where Gwen had hidden among the bushes and brambles surrounding the house, in order to catch a glimpse of her 'Master'.

Back in Britain, I visited the National Library of Wales in Aberystwyth, where Ceridwen Lloyd-Morgan has done such important work in making the Gwen John archive more accessible. Here I found other material, including Gwen's correspondence with her friend Ursula Tyrrwhitt. These letters are written in the voice of a mature woman, speaking as one artist to another, discussing work methods, exhibitions, her relationship with her family, the high cost of creativity – so different from the 'little girl' tones begging her 'Master' to visit more often.

At the National Museum of Wales in Cardiff I found Gwen John's sketchbooks. Here were the artist's doodles as well as the scrupulously executed pencil drawings. In her endless search for perfection Gwen spent hour upon hour meticulously copying a small prayer card or experimenting with different tones. It was impossible not to be moved and impressed by her sheer determination and persistence, knowing of the many obstacles, both internal and external, that might have impeded her creative work.

I was later glad of the opportunity to discuss what I had seen with acknowledged experts, including Michael Holroyd, whose lively and detailed biography of Augustus John had given me many valuable insights into the relationship between brother and sister.

I also had a fascinating discussion with Mary Taubman; her excellent book *Gwen John* became my most valuable reference as well as providing me with easy access to the beautifully clear reproductions of most of the paintings mentioned in the play.

Discussions with practising artists were, of course, vital in helping me to understand more about techniques and materials. As a result I began to look at paintings with a more informed and critical eye.

But throughout the entire process of writing the play my most significant point of reference and source of inspiration was Gwen herself. As she spoke to me through her paintings, in her distinctive, quiet, persistent voice, I felt that she and I were involved, as I have long been involved with other creative women, in a lively, personal and often acutely painful dialogue.

The play takes place in one room because that is, I believe, how women live, juggling love, faith, work, family, friendships, past and present, trying to make some sense of them all. I did most of the writing in my caravan in Devon, which is my nearest equivalent to Gwen's wooden shack.

The present text has emerged out of several drafts and as a result of the very creative and exciting rehearsal process leading to its first production at Theatr Clwyd in 1987. It owes a great deal to the care and commitment of Annie Castledine, who commissioned it, nurtured it, championed it and, of course, directed it.

I called the play *Self Portrait* because I make no secret of the fact that it is both biography and autobiography. I wrote it for my friends — women who are trying, often against appalling odds, to do creative work. May they have the strength and courage to persevere, as Gwen John did. May their work flourish and receive the recognition it deserves.

Sheila Yeger
Bristol, 1990

# ACKNOWLEDGEMENTS

Respectful thanks to my teacher, Ven. Geshé Damchö Yonten, whose compassion and wisdom are always a source of inspiration.

Special thanks to the following people who were so generous with their time, insights and expert advice: David Fraser Jenkins at the Tate Gallery; Michael Holroyd (also for the loan of the John Quinn letters); Ceridwen Lloyd-Morgan at the National Library of Wales; Diane Setch at the National Museum of Wales; Mary Taubman. Also to the sculptor Alain Ayers, for his advice on Rodin. And to Jan Shannon, who so ably translated the Rodin letters.

Thanks also to: Madame Hélène Pinet at the Musée Rodin; Robin Vousden at the Anthony d'Offay Gallery; staff at the Ashmolean and Bodleian in Oxford; Gillian Doël at the Norwich School of Art; Amanda Hopkinson; Sue James; the late Romilly John; and to Maureen Pickles, who typed the manuscript.

I am very much indebted to Ben and Sara John for the use of extracts from Gwen John's journal and from her letters to Ursula Tyrrwhitt, Auguste Rodin and others.

Special thanks to artists Dilys Banham, Stella Pole and Sue Hakes for their advice and friendship; to David and Paddy Price Hughes, who have given me a place to work; to my parents and sister; and to Rob Preece, who helped me to understand.

To my friends Coral Howard, Gilly Fraser and Pat V.T. West for endless cups of tea, criticism and support, but most of all for their courage.

And to Roger Stennett, and my sons, Ben and Sam, for their tolerance, good humour and support at all times.

Last, but not least, thanks to Annie Castledine, without whom there would be no *Self Portrait*.

Sheila Yeger
Bristol, 1990

# SELECT BIBLIOGRAPHY

*Gwen John* Mary Taubman (Scolar Press, 1985)

*Gwen John 1876–1939* Susan Chitty (Hodder & Stoughton, 1981)

*The Obstacle Race* Germaine Greer (Picador, 1979)

*Women Artists* Karen Petersen and J. J. Wilson (The Women's Press, 1978)

*Modern English Painters* Sir John Rothenstein (Eyre & Spottiswoode, 1952)

*Augustus John* Michael Holroyd (Heinemann, 1974, 1975, Penguin, 1976)

*Gwen John , an Interior Life* Cecily Langdale and David Fraser Jenkins (Phaidon Press and Barbican Art Gallery, 1985)

Gwen John papers at the National Library of Wales: Ceridwen Lloyd-Morgan

**Catalogues**
Mary Taubman: Introduction to the catalogue for the Faerber and Maison exhibition, 1964 and the Anthony d'Offay exhibition, 1976.

Augustus John: Foreword to the catalogue for the Gwen John memorial exhibition at the Matthiesen Gallery, London, 1946.

Michael Holroyd: Introduction to the catalogue for the Anthony d'Offay exhibition, 1982.

A. D. Fraser Jenkins: Foreword to the catalogue for the National Museum of Wales exhibition, 1976.

Sir John Rothenstein: Essay on Gwen John in the catalogue for the Tate Gallery and Arts Council exhibition, London, 1952.

**Unpublished Sources**
Musée Rodin, Paris: Letters from Gwen John to Auguste Rodin.

National Library of Wales, Aberystwyth: Miscellaneous letters, notebooks and diaries.

Tate Gallery, London: Miscellaneous letters.

New York Public Library: John Quinn correspondence.

Courtauld Institute, London: *Gwen John, her Art and her Religion* by Annela Twitchin, 1972.

*Self Portrait* was first presented at Theatr Clwyd by the Theatr Clwyd Company for Festival 1 on 23rd June 1987. It was directed by Annie Castledine with the following cast:

| | |
|---|---|
| GWEN JOHN: | Barbara Marten |
| BARBARA ROBSON: | Barbara Peirson |
| KAREN PITMAN and VERA OUMANÇOFF: | Stephanie Fayerman |
| MICHAEL LAWRENCE and JOHN QUINN: | Robert Pickavance |
| MOXI and DORELIA McNEILL: | Kim Hicks |
| SISTER MARY URSULA and A NUN: | Marlene Sidaway |
| FRANK WEBSTER and JACQUES MARITAIN: | Phil Rowlands |
| ROBERT LUCAS, AUGUSTUS JOHN, EDWIN JOHN and AUGUSTE RODIN: | Paul Humpoletz |
| PHILIPPA REYNOLDS, IDA JOHN and A YOUNG NUN: | Karen Gledhill |

Designer: Jenny Blincow
Choreographer: Duncan Holt
Lighting Designer: Keith Hemming
Sound: Vernon Nelson
Original music by Anthea Gomez

The play was subsequently presented at the Derby Playhouse on 1st June 1990. It was directed by Annie Castledine with the following cast:

| | |
|---|---|
| GWEN JOHN: | Lucinda Curtis |
| BARBARA ROBSON: | Deidra Morris |
| KAREN PITMAN and VERA OUMANÇOFF: | Stephanie Fayerman |
| MICHAEL LAWRENCE and JOHN QUINN: | Stefan Escreet |
| MOXI and DORELIA McNEILL: | Kim Hicks |
| SISTER MARY URSULA and A NUN: | Pauline Jefferson |
| FRANK WEBSTER and JACQUES MARITAIN: | Peter Meakin |
| ROBERT LUCAS, AUGUSTUS JOHN, EDWIN JOHN and AUGUSTE RODIN: | Robert Pickavance |
| PHILIPPA REYNOLDS, IDA JOHN and A YOUNG NUN: | Susan Gardner |

Designer: Steve Richardson
Movement: Duncan Holt
Musician: Clare David
Lighting: Nick Beadle
Sound: Alison Thorpe

# CHARACTERS

GWEN JOHN
AUGUSTUS JOHN: her brother
EDWIN JOHN: her father
IDA JOHN (née Nettleship): first wife of Augustus
DORELIA McNEILL: Augustus's lover (later his wife)
AUGUSTE RODIN
JOHN QUINN: Gwen John's American patron
JACQUES MARITAIN: Catholic philosopher
VERA OUMANÇOFF: Maritain's sister-in-law
TWO NUNS AT DIEPPE

BARBARA ROBSON: a novelist, about 40
KAREN PITMAN: exhibition organiser, about 40
MICHAEL LAWRENCE: owner of the Lawrence Art Gallery, late 40's
FRANK WEBSTER: a journalist, about 40
ROBERT LUCAS: a writer and television personality, 50's
PHILIPPA REYNOLDS: Robert's lover, early 20's
MOXI: an art student, about 20
SISTER MARY URSULA: a nun, 50's

# NOTES

The text of the tape used in the production was largely drawn from the video on Gwen John made by the ILEA Resources Centre.

The paintings referred to in the text may mostly be found in Mary Taubman's book *Gwen John*.

'Ben Bolt': words by Thos. Dunn English, melody by Nelson Kneass.

# ACT ONE

*An elegant art gallery. A banner proclaims:— 'Gwen John:
1876–1939'. A number of her paintings, amongst them, 'Self
Portrait in a Red Blouse' (Taubman Plate 11) and 'Mère Poussepin'
(Taubman Plate 40). A scrubbed pine table in front of a casement
window with a full-length white lace curtain. On the table a small
glass containing primroses and blue polyanthus. S. R. of the table
a light-coloured wicker chair with a white cushion. Elsewhere, a
couch, a small sculpture which is the figure of a naked woman, a
pile of canvases, a stand with drawings. A small low round table
with a pile of glossy catalogues, an antique box, a writing-case. A
telephone, a hatstand, a full-length gilt mirror. A tape recorder
and slide projector with a screen for the slides.*

*KAREN, a woman of about 40, runs the tape to make sure it's in
working order. She is smartly dressed to look businesslike, in a
well-cut calf-length dark skirt, a crisp shirt and cravat. Her
manner is confident, sharp, cool.*

*The voice on the tape is that of a man, very cultured, easy on the ear.*

TAPE: "The war in Europe was just beginning in September
1939 when a frail elderly woman took the train to
Dieppe. There she collapsed and was taken to hospital,
where she died . . ."

> [KAREN *stops the tape and runs it fast forward. Several
> slides flash onto the screen in quick succession. They include a
> portrait of the John family, a picture of* AUGUSTUS JOHN,
> *'The Beach at Tenby', and the 'Self Portrait in a Red
> Blouse'.* KAREN *then runs the tape back. Enter* MICHAEL
> LAWRENCE. *He carries a tray on which there are glasses of
> red and white wine. He is an urbane man in his 40's, well-
> dressed but with a carefully contrived air of the eccentric. He
> puts the tray down and goes over to* KAREN. *He seems anxious.*]

KAREN: The tape's fine. Everything in working order.

MICHAEL: But . . .

> [KAREN *smiles.*]

KAREN: It wasn't plugged in.

> [*Pause.* MICHAEL *kisses* KAREN *extravagantly on the cheek.*]

MICHAEL: Karen, you're a genius!

> [KAREN *crosses to help herself to a glass of wine. She takes
> a sip.* MICHAEL *watches.*]

I decided against the Chablis. Thought it might look a little flashy. Mustn't offend the Sister Superior. Apparently she's just back from a stint in Calcutta . . .

KAREN: I thought you were joking when you said we ought to invite a nun.

MICHAEL: Well, she *did* paint seven of them.

KAREN: Where did you find her?

MICHAEL: Yellow Pages. Where else? Looked it up under 'Mercy, Sisters of'. I shall ask Webster to get a snap of her in front of 'Mère Poussepin'. [*indicates the painting*] Sort of wimple to wimple.

KAREN: You'd better make sure he doesn't drink as much as he did last time, or the only thing he'll get a snap of is the inside of the gents' loo . . .

[*She goes over to the pile of catalogues and tidies up.
MICHAEL wanders around in a fidgety way, half looking at the pictures. KAREN watches him.*]

What do you *really* think of them?

MICHAEL: Technically, they're quite brilliant.

KAREN: But you don't like them.

MICHAEL: One can't help admiring them . . .

KAREN: If only they weren't so small.

MICHAEL: You must admit she *did* tend to work in miniature.

KAREN: So did Jane Austen.

[*The phone rings. KAREN goes to answer it. She picks up the receiver. We hear the pips at the other end. KAREN looks alarmed.*]

Barbara . . . where the hell are you? Where? [*Pause.*] . . . No, of course I didn't know it was raining . . . [*Pause.*] Look, I can't talk now . . . [*Pause.*] Because we've got a private view . . . [*Pause.*] Gwen John . . . John . . . [*spells*] J-O-H-N . . . [*sighs*] She was the sister of Augustus . . .

[*MICHAEL signals "Who is it?"*]

. . . I don't think that would be a good idea, I really don't . . . [*Pause.*] Because I'm working, that's why . . . [*Pause.*] Barbara, don't be so absurd . . . they're not worth it, any of them, especially not *him*. [*Pause.*] Oh, for God's sake, Barbara . . .

[*Enter MOXI, an art student. She is about 20, dark, ragged, beautiful, with a wild, gypsy-like quality. She wears a long black dress trimmed at the neck with white and a floppy red bow. (Taubman Plate 15). She carries an easel and a Moses basket. In the basket there are boxes and tubes of paints, a*]

*china palette, pencils, charcoal, brushes, a number of small
canvases and a baby.* MICHAEL, *very alarmed, rushes up to
her.*]

MICHAEL: I'm terribly sorry . . . I think there must be some . . .
[MOXI, *unperturbed, puts down the basket and begins to
unload the materials.*]

MOXI: I was told to ask for Karen . . . um . . .

MICHAEL: Pitman? Miss Pitman is on the — er . . .
[*He gestures desperately at* KAREN.]

KAREN: [*on the phone*] I can't talk now . . .

MOXI: She phoned the Slade. Said a 3rd year, preferably
female. Complete with easel. Add a touch of colour,
she said . . .

KAREN: [*on the phone*] If you promise you won't . . .
[*The money runs out.*]
Oh damn . . .
[*She puts the phone down.* MICHAEL *comes rushing over,
gesturing at* MOXI *and all her belongings.* MOXI *begins to
wander round, looking at the pictures in a sort of daze.*]

MOXI: They're amazing . . . Here's that one of her room in
Paris . . . the tones are incredible . . . the paint's as
thick as mud.
[*She looks at the painting very closely then reaches out to
touch it almost reverently.*]
Naples yellow, I'd say . . . black, vermilion . . . crimson
. . . yes, definitely Naples yellow . . . By the way . . . I'm
Moxi . . . short for Moxibustion . . . it's something to
do with burning. And this . . . [*indicates the baby*] . . . is
Daisy Star. [*to* KAREN] Ten pounds, you said. And all
the wine I could drink.

MICHAEL: [*to* KAREN] Who was that on the phone?
[KAREN *tries to look nonchalant.*]

KAREN: Just a friend. I told her to pop in. I hope that's O.K.

MICHAEL: Journalist, is she?

KAREN: Afraid not. Actually, she's writing a novel.
[*She gives him a big smile and exits.*]

[*Enter* SISTER MARY URSULA. *She is a robust-looking
woman in her 50's. She wears a traditional nun's habit.*
MOXI *jumps visibly.* SISTER MARY URSULA *approaches*
MICHAEL.]

SISTER: Are you Mr. Michael Lawrence? [*extends her hand*] Sister
Mary Ursula.

MICHAEL: Can I get you a coffee?

SISTER:     No, thank you, I've had my tea. [*looks around*] Are these the paintings? [*moves to study one more closely*] So much pain. A soul crying out in torment. [*notices the wine*] Well, perhaps a very small glass of the white. Since it *is* so freely offered.

[*She smiles hugely.* MICHAEL *hands her a glass of wine.*]

[*Enter* KAREN.]

KAREN:      No sign of Frank Webster . . . or any of the other hacks.

[MICHAEL *looks at his watch.*]

He's probably trying to decide whether the prospect of free booze *ad infinitum* is sufficient to offset the tedium of yet another 'minor artist', a woman to boot. [*parodies*] "These delicate little pictures in no way as dramatic as those of her more famous brother . . ."

MICHAEL:    You know, Karen, sometimes you are in danger of being a tiny bit boring.

KAREN:      Perish the thought . . . I think I'll start the tape.

[*She goes to the tape recorder and sets it going.* SISTER MARY URSULA *wanders over to listen.* MICHAEL *replenishes the white wine.* MOXI *studies the 'Self Portrait' very closely and then begins to prepare her palette. She sets up her easel. Throughout the play, she will work with great concentration, copying the portrait.*]

TAPE:       "The war in Europe was just beginning in September 1939 when a frail elderly woman took the train to Dieppe. There she collapsed and was taken to hospital, where she died. As she carried no belongings and no means of identification she was buried in an unmarked grave. Her name was Gwen John . . ."

[*Slide: 'Self Portrait in a Red Blouse'.*]

AUGUSTUS:   [*voice on tape*] "She wasn't chaste or subdued but amorous and proud. She didn't steal through life but preserved a haughty independence which some people mistook for humility. Her passions, both for men and women, were outrageous and irrational . . ."

[*During this, enter* FRANK WEBSTER. *He is a journalist. In his mid 40's, he looks more than a little frayed around the edges, as if he is permanently running behind time.* KAREN *goes over to him and hands him a catalogue. He takes it.*]

FRANK:      Just dashed back from Battersea. Drama critic called off and muggins had to fill in. Now, remind me, what is it I've come to pontificate about today?

KAREN:      [*pointing to the catalogue*] Gwen John. 1876 to 1939.

FRANK: Any relation to —?

KAREN: His sister.

> [FRANK *opens the catalogue and starts to flick through it in a desultory fashion then glances around.*]

Some people, including her brother, consider her the greater artist . . .

FRANK: Bit insipid for my taste . . .

> [KAREN *goes over to the wine and gestures 'red or white'?*]

Red please. Got to keep my strength up.

> [KAREN *brings him a glass.*]

I'm a Spencer man myself. Now that's what I call genius. A huge talent . . . massive. Such a . . . a *muscular* quality . . .

> [*He wanders off.* MICHAEL *sighs, long-suffering.*]

MICHAEL: I think I'll bring up another case of the white . . .

> [*He exits.*]

> [*The tape comes up.* KAREN *goes past* MOXI. *She looks at how she's progressing.*]

TAPE: ". . . in the shadow of her brother's massive reputation. But time would judge, as Augustus knew."

AUGUSTUS: [*voice on tape*] "In fifty years' time I shall be remembered as the brother of Gwen . . ."

> [*Slide: family picture.*]

TAPE: "Their early years were spent in the Welsh seaside town of Tenby. Edwin, their father, was a solicitor and Augusta, their mother, an amateur artist. She died when Gwen was eight."

> [*The sound of seagulls.*]

> [*Slide: 'The Beach at Tenby'.*]

"The bleak childhood, spent with the silent and unsympathetic parent . . ."

> [KAREN *stands next to* FRANK. FRANK *looks at his watch.* KAREN *sees this.*]

KAREN: Not rushing off, I hope?

> [FRANK *looks longingly at the door.*]

FRANK: Well . . .

KAREN: Of course, you know she had a passionate relationship with the sculptor, Rodin. She wrote to him three times a day . . .

> [FRANK *instantly brightens. He reaches into his pocket and pulls out a notebook.*]

FRANK: Letters, did you say? *Love* letters? How . . . explicit . . . are they?

KAREN:     Somewhat.

> [FRANK *starts to look around with renewed interest.*]

> [*Enter* MICHAEL *with* BARBARA. *She is a strongly individual-looking woman of about 40, dressed with a shabby panache. She is bedraggled and very angry. She wears a dark blue long coat, which is open, and carries a white umbrella. She is struggling to free herself from* MICHAEL *who has hold of her arm. Both are very agitated.*]

BARBARA:   [*overlapping*] For the last time, will you get your bloody hands off me . . . ?

MICHAEL:   [*overlapping*] I told you. This is a private view. By invitation only . . .

BARBARA:   [*seeing* KAREN] Karen. Kindly tell this fucking maniac . . .

> [*A ripple of disapproval.*]

KAREN:     Barbara!

> [*She almost runs towards her.* BARBARA *obviously expects an embrace but* KAREN *stops short.*]

> Look at the state of you.

BARBARA:   I told you . . . it was raining.

> [*Pause.*]

MICHAEL:   Am I to conclude that you two . . . are acquainted?

BARBARA:   We went to school together. The Convent of the Sacred Heart. Karen was Captain of Hockey. I was excused games because of excessive bleeding.

MICHAEL:   [*to* KAREN] The lady novelist, I presume.

KAREN:     [*to* MICHAEL] I'm sorry. She wouldn't take no for an answer.

MICHAEL:   Can I get you a coffee?

BARBARA:   I'd prefer a drink.

> [KAREN *looks at* MICHAEL *as if to say, "What can I do?" He raises his eyebrows and marches off, very peeved.* KAREN *half drags* BARBARA *to the table. She takes the umbrella and rests it against the wicker chair. She helps* BARBARA *out of her coat and puts it over the arm of the chair.*]

KAREN:     You'll get me the sack . . . [*looks at* BARBARA] You look terrible. What the hell have you been doing?

BARBARA:   Crying mostly. I've been doing rather a lot of crying.

KAREN:     Honestly Barbara, what *is* the point?

BARBARA:   That's what I wanted to ask *you.* What's the point of any of it? [*Pause.*] I'm supposed to be writing a book. At least I thought that was what I was doing . . . But I seem to be lost . . . Can't find a map. On the road to nowhere. I sit looking out of the window at the kids going to

school. Seven hours later, there they are, coming home
again. History, geography, language and literature.
And I haven't written a word. Not a single bloody word.

KAREN: I'd better get you a drink. Red or white?

BARBARA: Oh, definitely red. [*with vicious self-parody*] Red, the
colour of blood and salami. Red, the colour of raw liver
and self-sacrifice. Our first school dance, remember? I
desperately wanted a red dress. Red with a black sash.
Like Irma la Douce. Naturally, my mother said no! I
was to wear pink. Pink for a girl, said mother. Bet
you've forgotten the Gay Gordons . . .

> [*She starts to sing the tune and forces* KAREN *into a fierce
> lampoon of the dance.* KAREN *pulls free and tries to walk
> away.* BARBARA *grabs her.*]

Is *he* coming?

KAREN: Who?

BARBARA: Don't play games. You know who I mean. Robert
Lucas. *Is* he coming or isn't he?

KAREN: [*struggling to free herself*] Barbara, please. I don't know.
I've lost the list.

BARBARA: You're lying again. It's getting to be a bit of a habit . . .

KAREN: Look . . . perhaps it would be better if you . . .

BARBARA: Died? Swallowed my tongue? Saw a psychiatrist?

KAREN: Listen . . .

BARBARA: No, *you* listen. Yesterday I had a new felt tip pen. Black.
Very fine. I wrote my name. I wrote *his* name. I crossed
off the letters like we used to do at school. Love, Like,
Hate, Adore. Barbara adores Robert. Robert hates
Barbara. Was it 'hate' made him want to reach up
inside me, first one finger, then two, then three, then
four . . . ? Was it 'hate' as he lay beside me, his mouth
against my . . . ?

> [MICHAEL *comes in.*]

MICHAEL: Feeling better? Karen tells me you're writing a novel.
How absolutely fascinating.

> [BARBARA *laughs.*]

BARBARA: Fascinating? No, that's not the word. Bizarre, yes.
Presumptuous, maybe. Suicidal, definitely. It's as if
I've swallowed a stone and I'm forced to live with it
lodged in my gut . . . it's as if I'm pregnant and utterly
incapable of giving birth . . .

MICHAEL: It all sounds so terribly painful.

BARBARA: Yes.

[*At that moment* ROBERT LUCAS, *with* PHILIPPA REYNOLDS
(PIP) *in tow, makes a calculated dramatic entrance. He is in
his 50's, tall, bearded, very handsome, hoping to be
considered charismatic. He is flamboyantly well-dressed to
command the maximum attention. He wears a long black
cloak and large black hat, boots, gloves, and waistcoat and
carries a cane.* PIP *is in her 20's, quietly spoken, very pale,
with long brown hair. She wears a rather demure long skirt.*]

[MICHAEL *rushes towards* ROBERT.]

MICHAEL: [*to* KAREN] Fetch Mr. Lucas a drink.

[*He greets* ROBERT *effusively.*]

ROBERT: At last . . . How wonderful! [*looking round as if surveying his
creation*] How absolutely wonderful!

[*He takes off his hat and aims it at the hatstand. It misses.*
PIP *rushes to pick it up. She hangs it on the stand. He then
signals to her to take his cloak, which he has removed, also his
gloves and cane. She stands there looking awkward till*
KAREN *relieves her of them and puts them on the stand.
Everybody, including* BARBARA, *watches all this, as was
intended. Then* SISTER MARY URSULA *goes over to the tape
recorder. As she passes* BARBARA *she smiles warmly and
touches her arm.* BARBARA *isn't sure how to interpret this.
She too goes to the tape, but her eyes never leave* ROBERT.]

TAPE: ". . . a gregarious period in Gwen's life, spent among
her fellow students. Two are depicted here in a drawing
by Augustus: Ursula Tyrrwhitt, Gwen's lifelong friend
with whom she regularly corresponded, and Ida
Nettleship, Augustus's first wife."

[*Slide: drawing of Ursula Tyrrwhitt and Ida Nettleship.*]

[*Meanwhile,* ROBERT, PIP *beside him, looks around.* KAREN
*and* MICHAEL *hover.*]

KAREN: [*to* ROBERT] Do you know her work?

ROBERT: Of course! Doesn't everyone? After all, she *was* the
sister of . . .

KAREN: In the opinion of many, *including* Augustus, she was the
far superior artist.

MICHAEL: Karen tells me you were thinking of featuring the
exhibition on the programme . . .

ROBERT: It's a possibility. Of course, I would need to consult my
assistant . . .

[*He puts his arm round* PIP*'s shoulders.*]

Have you met Pip . . . ? Sorry . . . *Philippa* Reynolds?

MICHAEL: Reynolds, eh! Now *there's* a name . . .
> [PIP *looks blank. They shake hands.*]

ROBERT: Pip's my right-hand man these days, aren't you, sweetheart? Dare not take a step without her.
> [BARBARA *seems to take a decision. She walks up to* ROBERT.]

BARBARA: Hallo, Robert.

KAREN: I think you may know Miss Robson.
> [ROBERT *gives an all-purpose smile.* BARBARA *exits with a fierce dignity.*]

MICHAEL: About the programme . . . Of course she *did* have a relationship with . . .
> [KAREN *looks daggers at him.*]

KAREN: The real motif of her work is the interaction of self and subject. There's this extraordinary intensity, a sort of obsessiveness almost . . .
> [ROBERT *stifles a yawn, smiles at* PIP *and squeezes her hand.*]

Her control of the medium really is remarkable. There's always this powerful combination of passion and technique. And she only painted women, or subjects close to her. The people she saw in church, children in Brittany, her room in Paris, her cats . . .
> [ROBERT'*s eyes focus on* BARBARA *who has just come in again.*]

ROBERT: A relationship with who?
> [KAREN *sighs, defeated.*]

KAREN: Rodin.

ROBERT: We might be able to use *that.* [*to* PIP] What do you think, poodle? [*smiles*] I call her poodle. I've always loved that marvellously erotic thing he did . . .

KAREN: 'The Kiss' . . .

ROBERT: Well, it's certainly worth a thought . . . [*sees* WEBSTER] Frank, my dear chap, still wallowing in slime?
> [*They wander off together.* PIP *watches* BARBARA *for a moment then exits.*]
>
> [SISTER MARY URSULA *comes up to* MOXI, *who is still drawing.*]

SISTER: You draw well.

MOXI: I'm learning.

SISTER: We're all learning.

MOXI: It seems to take such a long time.
> [SISTER MARY URSULA *nods.*]

And things keep getting in the way.

[*The baby starts to cry.*]

See . . .

KAREN:  Moxi . . . If you want the Ladies . . .

[MOXI *picks up the baby in the basket and exits. The crying continues offstage.*]

[*In the following sequence* ROBERT *is seen as* AUGUSTUS JOHN *and* PIP *as* IDA JOHN.]

[*In this and subsequent sequences there is no change of costume. The characters in the present freeze or fade into the background. Except where specifically indicated, they show no awareness of or reaction to the characters from the past.*]

[*Enter* IDA JOHN, *carrying a great pile of nappies. She looks flustered and dishevelled. She looks around rather desperately for somewhere to put the nappies, then drops them on top of* MOXI's *palette. The baby cries on.*]

AUGUSTUS:  [*shouting, off*] Stop that bloody row, can't you?

[*The crying continues.* IDA *looks exasperated, then the picture on the easel catches her attention. She looks at it with an informed eye.*]

IDA:  Not bad. Not bad. In fact . . . rather good.

[*The baby cries on.* IDA *picks up a paintbrush and paints in the air as if conducting the screams.*]

AUGUSTUS:  [*shouting, off*] Shut up, I said. Some people are trying to do a bit of work!

[IDA *puts the brush down. She takes one of the nappies and puts it over her head.*]

[*shouting*] Ida. Ida!

[AUGUSTUS JOHN *thunders into the scene. He is a large man, aged 24, very flamboyant. He carries a large brush dripping red paint.*]

I think I may go mad!

[*He plucks the nappy off* IDA's *head and uses it to clean his brush, then drops it on the floor.* IDA *picks it up, surveys the red paint on it, then folds it and returns it to the pile. The baby cries on.* AUGUSTUS *shouts over it.*]

A baby, you said. Doting little eyes gazing up at me . . . "Dadda, dadda." My first-born son. Looking up to his father for inspiration and guidance. Following in the paternal footsteps . . . flesh of my flesh! [*Pause.*] No one ever warned me about *screaming*. I ask you, Ida, how is a man supposed to paint a masterpiece to the constant sound of "Waaa"?

[*Suddenly the baby stops screaming. They look at one another, disbelieving. After a moment, enter* GWEN JOHN. *She is 26 years old, dressed as in the 'Self Portrait', minus the shawl. She is physically small, very self-contained, with an air of unusual intensity and fierce determination. She speaks softly, with precision, with a trace of a Pembrokeshire accent. She strides purposefully to the pile of nappies and disentangles the palette. Then she crosses to the painting and touches it with the tip of her finger.* IDA *watches her.*]

IDA: It's dry. I just looked.

GWEN: Good.

[*She examines her palette.*]

IDA: It's the best thing you've done so far. Better than anything you did at the Slade. The colours are brilliant. Don't you think so, Gus?

[GWEN *glances at* AUGUSTUS *but he is pacing about, distracted. She begins to paint onto the canvas. She works with great absorption.* IDA *watches.*]

You went to the baby. Thanks.

GWEN: I sang him a song.

IDA: Which one?

GWEN: 'Ben Bolt'. He seemed to like the chorus.

[*She sings a little.* IDA *laughs.* AUGUSTUS *suddenly stops pacing about and sits down heavily on the pile of nappies, head in hands.* IDA *and* GWEN *exchange glances.*]

AUGUSTUS: I may go out.

[IDA *and* GWEN *carefully fail to react.*]

I can't stay cooped up here all day. I need stimulation . . . space . . . freedom to be myself.

[*He strides over to the painting and looks at it.*]

Ida's right. It's bloody good. My gifted little sister!

[*He goes to the hatstand, puts on the cloak and picks up the hat.*]

I suppose it's for the Slade Show.

GWEN: [*suddenly less certain*] I don't really know. I may not be finished in time. [*stands back, surveys it*] I'm not sure whether I've succeeded with the blouse. I may have to start again.

AUGUSTUS: I said it was good, didn't I? Not that my opinion counts for anything round these parts.

[GWEN *paints on.*]

IDA: Are you entering anything, Gus?

AUGUSTUS: From among my current masterpieces, you mean?

Portrait of the artist under siege . . . portrait of the artist as a family man . . . self portrait surrounded by shit? Oh, I'll enter. You know me! Man's got a reputation to keep up. The great and glorious . . . the undoubtedly underestimated . . . I give you . . . Augustus John . . .

[*He whirls around with the cloak, very dramatic.*]

IDA: Poor Gus . . . I'm so sorry . . .

[*She runs to him, mothers him.*]

AUGUSTUS: What the hell are you apologising for?

IDA: Being alive, I suppose.

· [*The baby starts to cry again.* IDA *and* AUGUSTUS *look at each other. Then* IDA *exits.*]

GWEN: Why do you keep hurting her?

AUGUSTUS: Mind your own business, dear sister. Married bliss — hardly your province, is it?

GWEN: Sometimes it's hard to keep quiet.

[AUGUSTUS *goes to the canvas and stabs at it with his finger.*]

AUGUSTUS: Painting. That's what you're good at. Alarmingly good, actually. Stick to painting and leave life to the rest of us.

[*He exits.* GWEN *watches him go.*]

GWEN: So much pain.

[GWEN *moves so that she is standing behind* BARBARA. BARBARA *is looking at a painting. Seeming to sense something, she turns. For a moment they are almost face to face.*]

BARBARA: [*to herself*] How does anyone ever learn to bear the pain?

[GWEN *wanders off among the paintings.* MOXI *comes back in. She stands looking critically at what she has achieved so far.* FRANK *crosses to join her.*]

FRANK: How are *you* getting along?

MOXI: I think it's a bit of a mess. [*points to the original*] It's all these layers and glazes. She makes it look so easy, but, believe me, it isn't . . .

FRANK: [*looking at* MOXI's *effort*] Better than I could do, anyhow.

MOXI: Are you an artist?

[FRANK *guffaws.*]

FRANK: No, I'm just a humble pen-pusher.

MOXI: Oh, you're a writer.

FRANK: Not so you'd notice. I'm a mere journalist. A creature of the gutter. [*Pause.*] What are you doing afterwards? Fancy a steak? There's a Berni just round the corner.

MOXI: I don't eat meat.

FRANK: Oh, one of them! Bet you don't drink either. Or do the other thing. God, I hate the younger generation. They're so blameless it makes you want to vomit. What *do* you do, eh?

MOXI: I paint and I look after Daisy Star.

FRANK: Who the hell's . . . ? [*sees the baby*] Oh . . . that . . . Still, you could do with a bit of feeding up . . . you're wasting away. Bit like little Miss John here . . . too bloody skinny by half. You sure I can't tempt you to a steak . . . a nut cutlet . . . a kidney bean casserole . . . ?

[GWEN *stands by the tape recorder.*]

TAPE: " . . . was later to develop this sense of tone and methodical technique to the point of elaboration, preparing her own canvases and colour mixes and inventing a system of numbering her tones . . ."

GWEN: [*voice on tape*] "Sky 22 . . . Clouds 13 . . . Faded Roses 3 reds . . ."

TAPE: "Back in London, she was again in her brother's circle. In his dynamic and complicated world, Gwen was stifled. Her escape was made with Dorelia McNeil, Augustus's lover."

[*Slide: 'Dorelia in a Black Dress' (Taubman Plate 15).*]

"Their destination was Rome but they only succeeded in reaching Toulouse . . ."

[GWEN *turns away from the slide.*]

GWEN: Dorelia . . . Dodo . . . Did you really think we'd ever get to Rome . . . ? Did it even matter *where* we got to . . . ? We were together . . . in the open air . . . free as birds . . . nothing to stop us . . . nobody to tell us what to do. Only the sky and the hedges and we could lie awake all night and draw all day . . . Dodo . . .

[*She wanders over to the small table and picks up the writing case and a pen. She carries it to the pine table, sits, and begins to write.*]

[MOXI *comes in as* DORELIA. *She approaches* GWEN *and puts her arms round her from behind.* GWEN *turns and kisses her on the mouth.*]

DORELIA: Writing to Ursula?

GWEN: Yes.

DORELIA: [*reading over* GWEN*'s shoulder from the letter*] "You would like this place. It is very artistic. The country round is wonderful, especially now. The trees are all colours. I

paint my picture on the top of a hill . . . I cannot tell you
how wonderful it is when the sun goes down. The last
two evenings have had a red sun . . . 'lurid', I think is
the word. The scene is sublime then — it looks like Hell
or Heaven." [*Pause.*] You know, you should have been a
writer. You have a way with words.

GWEN: [*getting up*] You mean, more than with paint?

DORELIA: Would I say that?

> [*She goes to look at the painting on the easel.*]

It's . . . well . . . it's . . . coming on.

GWEN: [*going to look at it*] It's terrible.

DORELIA: If I had a pound for every time I've heard you say that
. . . You make such ridiculous demands on yourself.

> [*She touches GWEN's hair.*]

I prefer your hair loose. It makes you look more . . .
[*searches for the word*] . . . free.

> [*GWEN moves away from her, agitated.*]

GWEN: Shall we start? While there's still some light?

DORELIA: Work. I almost forgot.

GWEN: It's what we came for.

DORELIA: Is it?

> [*DORELIA rather reluctantly takes up the pose. (Taubman
> Plate 15). GWEN stands at the easel and looks at DORELIA.*]

GWEN: The hands are too low.

> [*DORELIA adjusts her hands. GWEN is still dissatisfied. She
> goes across to DORELIA and shifts her hands by a fraction of
> an inch then stands back and squints at her.*]

There's still something wrong.

> [*She adjusts the pose again and stands back.*]

Sorry . . . you must feel like a sack of coal.

DORELIA: It's always like that when you model.

GWEN: Even when you model for the great Augustus John?

DORELIA: Especially.

> [*They laugh. GWEN begins to prepare her palette.*]

GWEN: Sometimes I wonder . . . Will we ever be as good as the
men? Those wonderful old masters . . . and the modern
men too. At college I used to look at them all . . . so full
of it always. They seem so enormous. Almost as if they
might swell up and occupy the whole world . . . as if
we'd better move fast before they take over everything
and there's no space left for us and our little bits of
work. The trouble is, the thought of it makes us hurry
. . . [*looks up*] Can you open your eyes very slightly . . . ?

You look a bit too modest.

[DORELIA *laughs and abandons the pose.*]

Please, Dodo . . . the light's going.

[DORELIA *reorganises herself.*]

DORELIA: Sorry . . . it was the thought of modesty.

[GWEN *goes over and adjusts the bow on* DORELIA*'s dress then returns to the easel. A long pause.*]

GWEN: Do you ever think of Ida? How she feels?

DORELIA: Ida doesn't mind about me. Not one little bit. Anyway, artists aren't like normal people . . . she must have known that when she married Gus. Gus says every great artist has either starved in a garret or had a string of mistresses . . . sometimes both . . . it's all part of the mystique, he says.

GWEN: You're talking rubbish as usual. Dangerous rubbish at that. Anyway . . . none of that interests me in the slightest. Work. That's the only thing. If the men want to play at being artists, let them. But if we women want to be taken seriously, we have to regard ourselves with the utmost seriousness.

[DORELIA *yawns hugely then laughs.*]

DORELIA: Sorry.

[GWEN *puts down her brush.*]

GWEN: Evidently you find this all a little tedious. .

DORELIA: I thought art would be fun.

GWEN: Then you thought wrong. Stand still, for God's sake.

[DORELIA *wanders over to look at the painting.*]

DORELIA: You make me look really wanton.

[GWEN *looks at her, then back to the painting.* DORELIA *still stares at it, fascinated, then she coils up her hair with her hand, in a rather provocative gesture. Suddenly she snatches* GWEN*'s paintbrush and sticks it in her hair, then she runs off, brandishing it, laughing wildly.* GWEN *runs after her, catches her, holds her. Both are laughing. Freeze. Then* DORELIA *runs off.*]

GWEN: Dodo . . . Dodo . . . don't leave, not yet. He took you away . . . But it was all my own doing . . . I told you to go . . . How could I hold you . . . ? It was like trying to hold a wild animal . . . like a part of myself I must always hold in check . . . in case . . . in case . . . [*Pause.*] I wanted to get it right. All of it. I always wanted so badly to get it right.

[*Light on* ROBERT *as* EDWIN JOHN. *He harangues* GWEN *across the room.*]

EDWIN: Worse than a common prostitute. My own daughter . . . the daughter of Edwin John . . . not content with running off with a common little typist, making me the laughing stock of all Tenby, sleeping, as I understand it, in the *open air*, begging for food . . .

GWEN: We did *not* beg. We drew portraits of people and sold them . . .

EDWIN: No better than gypsies.

GWEN: There is nothing wrong with gypsies, Papa. Ask Gussy. He . . .

EDWIN: Don't argue with me, young woman. Consorting with . . .

GWEN: It wasn't an argument. I merely . . .

EDWIN: All the riff-raff . . . the rag-tag-and-bobtail . . . Fearing as any father would for your well-being . . .

GWEN: I told you, Father . . . I am perfectly . . .

EDWIN: Full of trepidation for your welfare . . . wishing only to offer you moral support . . .

GWEN: I have no need for your support, moral or . . .

EDWIN: Prepared to forgive and forget . . . at considerable expense and no little inconvenience . . . I find you installed in a room which one would hesitate to offer a scullery maid, yet merry as anything . . . in no way repentant . . . showing no sign of contrition . . . and, what is more, displaying your . . . your *self* in a dress which would not look out of place in what do they call it . . . the Follies . . . the Follies . . .

GWEN: Bergère. Actually it is a copy of a gown depicted by Manet. I could show you the picture if you like.

EDWIN: A little drawing . . . yes. A decent enough accomplishment for a woman. Landscapes . . . flowers . . . portraits of suitable subjects. But this . . . this has gone too far.

[*The light goes off* EDWIN.]

[BARBARA *stands looking a the slide of* DORELIA. ROBERT *moves across to stand behind her. He kisses her on the back of the neck. She turns to face him.*]

BARBARA: You said you'd phone when you got back from Venice.

ROBERT: Did I?

BARBARA: I waited by the phone every day for a week. When I had to go out to get some bread I took the phone off the hook so that if you *did* call, you'd think it was engaged . . .

ROBERT:    You're not supposed to take it off the hook, Barbara. You're a very naughty girl. [*Pause.*] How are you, anyway? You look . . . *amazing.*

BARBARA:   I look like a witch.

ROBERT:    It could be that I am drawn to witches. How's the book? Finished it yet?

BARBARA:   There isn't a book. There won't be a book. It was crazy to even think I could do it. Women like me don't write books. They listen to men talking about books *they've* written.

ROBERT:    You really are looking rather extraordinary. All sort of dark and elegiac. Is it a new sort of cosmetic you've discovered?

BARBARA:   It's called insomnia. I lie awake at night listening to the lorries on the North Circular. I want to hate you but I seem to have lost the knack.

ROBERT:    I'm glad about that. Nobody likes to be hated.
           [*Pause.*]

BARBARA:   *Why* didn't you ring?

ROBERT:    Because I had a publisher's deadline to meet. Oh Barbara, I wish you wouldn't be so . . .

ROBERT:    What's her name?

ROBERT:    Who?

BARBARA:   Milly-Molly-Mandy. Your latest acquisition.

ROBERT:    Her name's Philippa, but she prefers to be called 'Pip'. She's the new P.A. on the programme.

BARBARA:   What's she like in bed?

ROBERT:    She's very amenable.

BARBARA:   Is that supposed to be in her favour?

ROBERT:    It does tend to make life a lot easier.

BARBARA:   Whose life, Robert? Whose life?
           [*Pause.* ROBERT *reaches out to touch the corner of* BARBARA's *eye.*]

ROBERT:    I love it when you get angry. It makes your eyes blaze up like bonfires. Oh, come here, will you . . . ?
           [*Looking around to make sure the coast is clear, he pulls her towards him.* GWEN *walks in and stands near them.*]
           You still want me, don't you?

BARBARA:   What?

ROBERT:    In spite of all your principles.

[*He starts to kiss her. At first she responds, then suddenly
breaks away.* GWEN *wanders off.*]

What's going on . . . ?

BARBARA: [*looking round*] I . . . don't know. [*shudders*] I don't
know . . .

[ROBERT *moves off a little. He takes out a small comb and
combs his beard.*]

ROBERT: [*putting away the comb*] What do you think of all this lot,
anyway? Bit wishy-washy for my taste.

BARBARA: I think they're . . . I think they're incredibly courageous.

ROBERT: Courageous?

BARBARA: Yes.

[*He looks at her, puzzled.* BARBARA *wanders off, still
obviously disturbed. A little off balance,* ROBERT *starts to
look idly through some drawings in a folder.* GWEN *appears
behind him. When he turns, it is as* EDWIN JOHN.]

GWEN: I see you've been looking at some of my pictures.

EDWIN: Just passing the time. Still . . . they're not bad. Bit
wishy-washy for my taste. But not bad. Your brother's
been doing some fine stuff lately. Nice and bright. Big
too. I like a picture that cheers you up. Shall we go to
the Eiffel Tower? Can't go back to Tenby without
having seen the Eiffel Tower.

[*Pause.*]

GWEN: Father, why don't you ever discuss my work?

EDWIN: I told you . . . they're nice little pictures. [*barely pausing*]
I should like to try some of those croissants they talk
about. Do you know where we can buy some?

GWEN: I usually make do with bread. It's cheaper and it goes
further.

EDWIN: Don't you start accusing me over money, young lady.
We've had all this out before. You *wanted* to live like this
— it's your own choice. You could easily come back to
England, settle down and open a little school or
something. Teach kiddies to draw. I'd give you every
encouragement and I'm sure your brother would too.
But madam prefers to starve herself to death in Paris,
pretending to be an artist.

[*A pause while* GWEN *attempts to absorb all this. She is
furious as well as desperately hurt.*]

GWEN: Why *did* you come?

EDWIN: Aren't you pleased to see me?

GWEN: I asked you why you had come.

EDWIN:   You're my daughter. A father likes to keep an eye. Anyway, Augustus said you'd been a little . . . what shall we say . . . ?

GWEN:    I've been ill.

EDWIN:   Nothing serious, I hope.

GWEN:    No. Nothing serious.

EDWIN:   You don't eat enough . . . and I'm sure you don't wear a vest. I'll never forget that ridiculous dress. It's no wonder you catch cold!

GWEN:    I'm trying to paint.

> [EDWIN *wanders over to the window. He parts the curtain and peers out.*]

EDWIN:   Not much of a view. Chimneys . . . rooftops . . .

GWEN:    Why don't you ever listen to me? I might as well be talking to myself.

> [EDWIN *turns suddenly.*]

EDWIN:   I can't make you out. If you want the truth, I never could. I've tried to help you. I've fallen over backwards to accommodate you — all your strange ideas, your awkward little ways. And how do you repay me? With rudeness, with sullenness, with spite. You know, Gwendolen, sometimes . . . I am regretfully drawn to the conclusion that you have taken leave of your senses.

GWEN:    Sometimes, Father, when I see sanity, I think I prefer madness. We'd better go out.

> [*She walks to the door.*]

EDWIN:   At least your brother knows how to make a decent living . . . doing very nicely for himself is young Augustus. Very nicely. Exhibitions. Picture in the newspapers. Way of life not everyone's cup of tea, I'll grant you that . . .

GWEN:    Ida is dead. Perhaps Dorelia will last longer. There is a man in New York who seems interested in my work. His name is John Quinn. He has offered me money on a regular basis.

EDWIN:   Well, that's nice, isn't it? When someone shows a bit of interest. Specially financial. Can you climb up the Eiffel Tower or do you just look at it from down below?

GWEN:    You can climb it. You can climb right to the top.

EDWIN:   And what do you do when you get there, eh? *That's* what I'd like to know.

GWEN:    You have three choices, Father. One: You walk down

again. Two: You jump off and break your neck. Three:
You grow wings and see if you can fly.

[*Brief blackout. In the blackout* GWEN's *voice on tape is heard.*]

GWEN: [*voice on tape*] "Dear Ursula, I think if we are to do beautiful pictures, we ought to be free of family conventions and ties. I think the family has had its day, don't you? We don't go to Heaven in families now, but one by one. I have been thinking of painting a good deal lately. I think I shall do something good soon, if I am left to myself and not absolutely destroyed . . ."

[*Slide: 'Corner of the Artist's Room in Paris (With Flowers)' (Taubman Plate 22).*]

[*Slide: 'Cat (Edgar Quinet)' (Taubman Plate 20). This slide remains on the screen throughout the following sequence.*]

[GWEN *moves across to the easel. She sings the first verse of 'Ben Bolt'.*]

"Oh, don't you remember sweet Alice, Ben Bolt.
Sweet Alice with hair so brown.
She wept with delight when you gave her a smile.
And trembled with fear at your frown."

[*She stands by the easel, holding some drawing paper. She takes several different pencils out of a jar there before finding one to her satisfaction. Then she looks around for something to draw.*]

[*spoken, not sung*] "She wept with delight when you gave her a smile, and trembled with fear at your frown."

[*The whole of the following is addressed to the cat as she draws and paints her.*]

Now . . . do you think you could try to keep still for a change? If I promise not to arrange you.

[*She draws quickly, with confidence and intense concentration.*]

You can arrange a jug of flowers. I could even arrange Dorelia. But a cat is a law unto itself.

[*She stops drawing. She looks critically at what she has done then holds it up to show to the cat.*]

There . . . what do you think? [*Pause.*] The nose a little pointed? [*looks at the drawing*] You could be right . . . You are of course my sternest critic.

[*She resumes drawing, correcting what she has done.*]

Not my *sternest* critic. *I* am my sternest critic.

[*She pours some water from a pitcher into a small jar. She*

*returns to the drawing and, using watercolour, mixes some
paint on her palette and begins to apply a wash to the drawing.*]

It's just as well my father didn't offer me money.
Because, of course, I should have been forced to refuse.
But, don't worry . . . we shall get by. There's always a
demand for models, even if I am a little on the thin side.
[*Pause.*] *You* liked the dress, didn't you? You *said* you
liked it. Perfectly nice, you said . . . but perhaps it *was*
cut just a little low.

[*She sings, almost under her breath.*]

"In the old churchyard, in the valley, Ben Bolt,
In a corner obscure and alone,
They have fitted a slab of granite so grey,
And sweet Alice lies under the stone . . ."

[*Long pause as she paints.*]

Being around Gussy always made me feel weak —
almost as if I couldn't breathe. They're so *big*, the men,
bigger than us somehow. I feel as if they're all around
me — not just now — but reaching back to the Greeks,
the Romans — important, massive — so much to say
that always seems of such great relevance . . . so much
*push*. Take exhibitions . . . all that fearful pressure . . .
all the competition . . . *They* simply thrive on it, don't
they! But not us. We seem to need more space to
expand and grow at our own pace, more time just to
learn who we *are*. They seem to be born *knowing* . . .
[*sighs deeply*] Sometimes I think we should keep ourselves
apart — for safety . . . like ants that can easily be
crushed under mighty feet . . . [*Pause.*] Perhaps if I'd
had the dress made up in a different colour, something
not quite so . . . so *bold* . . . a pale colour . . . a pretty
colour . . . white . . . pink . . .

[*She studies the picture, seems dissatisfied.*]

Too far. One always seems to go too far.

[*She stands looking at the picture critically.*]

[BARBARA *stands looking at one of the paintings.* PIP
*approaches her.*]

PIP: It must be difficult to draw cats, don't you think?
BARBARA: No, not really. They're always sleeping. My cats could
sleep through an earthquake. Probably comes of
having a clear conscience and very little brain.

[*Pause.*]

PIP:     I saw you looking at Robert.

BARBARA: Is that a crime?

PIP:     Do you know him?

BARBARA: Only slightly.

PIP:     Was it a long time ago?

BARBARA: Several years . . . or months . . . or perhaps it was just a few days, I really can't remember.

PIP:     Not that I mind. What Robert did before he met me is *his* business entirely. I don't believe in being possessive about the past, do you? Of course, if he started anything now, *that* would be a different matter. [*laughs*] I'd probably murder him. We're deeply in love, Robert and I. Deeply.
         [*Pause.*]

BARBARA: I'm so sorry.

PIP:     Sorry? [*Pause.*] You're Barbara, aren't you? I saw one of your letters. [*Pause.*] Robert was right about you, that's for sure.
         [*Long pause.*]

BARBARA: I feel I'd like to hold you, protect you from harm. I'd like to warn you that you are in grave danger, to advise you to escape while you still have the strength. The only problem is my mouth seems to be full of stones. I think it's called jealousy.
         [*Pause.*]

PIP:     He didn't say you were crazy.
         [MICHAEL *and* KAREN *are by the telephone.*]

MICHAEL: What's Webster's reaction?

KAREN:   He doesn't know much about art, but he's rather taken with the little girl from the Slade. [*Pause.*] I don't think he's particularly enthralled.
         [MICHAEL *sighs and looks across at* BARBARA.]

MICHAEL: I trust your friend's behaving herself?

KAREN:   I shouldn't think so for one minute! It would be an alien concept.
         [BARBARA *stands looking at a picture of 'Mère Poussepin' (Taubman Plate 40).* SISTER MARY URSULA *joins her.*]

BARBARA: She looks so calm.

SISTER:  To tell you the truth, I thought she looked a little bilious. Probably the convent food. It has a tendency to be very indigestible.
         [*Long pause.*]

BARBARA: How do you survive it? I've always wondered.

SISTER: Oh, you get used to it! We seem to drink rather a lot of weak tea.
[*She laughs.*]

BARBARA: No, I mean . . .

SISTER: Oh . . . *that.* [*Pause.*] It's funny . . . nobody ever asks about the hours spent in silent prayer, the separation from family and friends, the endless physical work — scrubbing, mending, digging, cleaning. Sex — that's all anyone ever wants to know about. Sex, and how to do without it. [*laughs*] If I were to write a book, it'd be top of the best-sellers list tomorrow!
[*Pause.*]

BARBARA: *I'm* writing a book . . . a novel.

SISTER: How very brave. Is it autobiographical?

BARBARA: It's based on the story of King Lear.

SISTER: It *sounds* autobiographical.
[*Pause.*]

BARBARA: I've never considered religion.

SISTER: Most people don't.

BARBARA: As any kind of answer, I mean.

SISTER: Oh no, it's never an answer. Just a great many more questions . . . [*looks at the painting*] Why did she paint all these nuns?

BARBARA: It's probably in the catalogue.
[SISTER MARY URSULA *looks in the catalogue.*]

SISTER: I didn't realise she was a Catholic. It says here she was converted in 1912. She was commissioned to do the nuns by the Dominican Sisters of Charity in Meudon. Mère Poussepin here . . . [*points to the painting*] . . . was their founder. Apparently she painted seven versions, one for every room in the convent. How very interesting.
[*She reads on.*]

BARBARA: Was it hard?

SISTER: I would imagine the habit would be rather fiddly . . . [*looks up*] Oh, you mean . . . ? [*considers*] To begin with, yes. An exquisite torment. You think of very little else. It fills every crevice of your body, this acute longing, this sense of profound loss . . .

BARBARA: Then comes peace . . . isn't that what they say? The blessed love of God replaces the crippling love of man. Tell me that's what happens and I'll sign up tomorrow.

[SISTER MARY URSULA *smiles*.]

SISTER: Nothing so dramatic. You learn to redirect your energies. Your daily work becomes more powerful. Your prayer becomes more intense. You keep asking for strength and if you're lucky you find enough courage to continue. Just day by day. That's all.

BARBARA: It sounds a bit like being a writer.

SISTER: Will your novel be published?

BARBARA: I doubt it.

SISTER: You must never lose hope . . .

BARBARA: Why not? I seem to have lost almost everything else . . .

[SISTER MARY URSULA *takes* BARBARA's *hands and presses them in hers.* BARBARA *looks surprised that this is happening but, after a while, does not resist.*]

[FRANK WEBSTER *is talking on the phone. He is dictating copy.*]

FRANK: . . . thousands of letters, erotic, passionate, and very explicit, chart the tempestuous course of her relationship with the sculptor Rodin, famous for his massive erotic . . . no, I've used that . . . for his massive and sensuous work: 'The Kiss'. Miss John's paintings, limited as they are in scope and subject matter, are, nevertheless, quintessentially feminine and in no way comparable to the more . . .

[*He is cut off; he bangs angrily on the receiver rest.*]

Bloody phones.

[*He keeps banging. The sound becomes the sound of a hammer on stone. It grows heavy, loud, insistent, then it is broken into by a gentle tapping on an external door. After a while, the hammering stops. In the following sequences,* ROBERT *is seen as* AUGUSTE RODIN.]

RODIN: [*shouting, off*] Go to hell! Tell whoever it is to go to hell. I'm working.

[*The hammering starts again. After a brief pause the tapping is repeated, then stops.*]

GWEN: [*standing at the door*] I understand that Monsieur Rodin is seeking a model. My name is Miss John. Miss Gwendolen Mary John.

[RODIN *appears, striding towards* GWEN *like an old testament prophet. He is an imposing if elderly man, massive, craggy. He carries a sculpture tool.* GWEN *stands looking tiny, insignificant and petrified. She wears an outdoor coat and hat and carries a small bag.*]

I knocked several times before I could make anyone
hear. I'm sorry if I've come at the wrong time. I . . .
[RODIN *pokes at her chest with the sculpture tool.*]

RODIN:  Too thin.

GWEN:  I'm sorry. Perhaps I should try to eat more. There
never seems to be the time . . . or the money. Shall I
take my clothes off now?
[RODIN *laughs heartily.* GWEN *stands awkwardly, unsure
what is expected.* RODIN *turns her around with his hand,
studies her.*]

RODIN:  It's a good straight back. [*staring at her*] Why are you
shivering? Do you find it cold?

GWEN:  No . . . no . . . in fact suddenly I feel extremely warm.
[RODIN *continues to scrutinise her. She is disturbed by this.*]

RODIN:  You could begin by removing your coat.
[GWEN *takes off her coat.*]
And that absurd hat.
[GWEN *takes off her hat.* RODIN *takes her coat, hat and bag
and lets them drop to the ground. He evaluates her.
Embarrassed,* GWEN *covers herself with her hands but*
RODIN *moves them away from her body.*]
Now your skirt.
[GWEN *unfastens her skirt and lets it fall to the ground.*
RODIN *lifts her petticoat to look at her legs.*]
The legs are a good shape . . . Oh . . . and now the er . . .
[*He indicates her blouse.* GWEN *unbuttons it nervously, her
eyes on him.* RODIN *stands back and assesses her. This is
done very clinically, almost as if he were considering buying
a horse or a piece of furniture.*]
You have a perfectly adequate body. In fact, without
your clothes you look a good deal larger than I
expected.
[GWEN *wraps her arms around herself, very self-conscious.*]
Why are you hiding?

GWEN:  I'm sorry . . . I . . .

RODIN:  For the love of God, will you stop apologising . . .
[*Brief blackout. When the lights come up again* GWEN
*stands with her back to us, naked, in the pose of* RODIN*'s
'Whistler's Muse'. Her left leg is raised on a plinth and her
head is slightly inclined.* RODIN *works with clay on an
armature.*]
So . . . how is my little artist today? You are doing your
drawing as instructed, I trust . . . ?

GWEN: I try. But I'm afraid I don't always succeed. Things seem to get in the way.

RODIN: Things? What things? If you want to be an artist you must practise your craft. I'm not interested in excuses.

> [*Mortified*, GWEN *lets her head droop.* RODIN *picks up a pair of steel pincers and goes to her. He measures her upper arm and adjusts her head: all this in a very impersonal way. He goes back to the sculpture.*]

Remember . . . an artist's only credentials are his work. Talking about art will get you nowhere.

GWEN: I'm only a beginner . . . an amateur. You mustn't even waste your time.

RODIN: If *you* think your work is nothing, then that's what it'll be — nothing. An artist's work can only be as important as he himself considers it. If *you* don't value what you do, how the hell can you expect anyone else to?

> [*He takes a sip of water from a glass, then spits it at the clay: an almost contemptuous gesture. Some of it sprays* GWEN. *She moves.* RODIN *is furious.*]

And don't move. For the love of God, don't move!

> [*He works on, then stops abruptly.* GWEN *is suddenly very nervous.* RODIN *hands her her coat. She pulls it tightly round her.*]

GWEN: [*rather desperate*] Are we finished? Can I go home now?

RODIN: We are finished *work* and of course you can go, but I suspect that you don't really want to.

GWEN: Yes I do.

RODIN: Do you?

> [*He slips his hand inside the coat and touches her breasts. She gasps, pulls it tighter and looks around as if trying to escape either from him or from herself.*]

GWEN: I *must* go. Edgar Quinet will be waiting for supper . . .

RODIN: [*in mock horror*] Edgar Quinet? Don't tell me you have a jealous lover.

> [GWEN *laughs, relaxes a little.*]

GWEN: She *is* jealous, but she's not my lover. Edgar Quinet is my cat. I named her after the street where I live. She is also my cheapest model. I wouldn't want to annoy her.

> [RODIN *laughs hugely.*]

What do you find so funny?

> [RODIN *puts his arms around her in a bear-like hug.*]

RODIN: You . . . *you* are funny. Funny and also very, very serious. And beautiful, in your plain, Welsh, sort of way. So beautiful that I must come right inside you and find out what is there.

[*He reaches down to touch her. She makes a feeble attempt to stop him.*]

There is no need to pretend that you're shocked. I felt your skin just before. You are burning, my little one, burning.

[*He kisses her. At first she responds timidly, then more passionately.*]

See . . . see.

[*He kisses her again. This time she completely abandons herself to it.*]

GWEN: Yes . . . oh yes . . . please . . . yes . . .

[*She begins to kiss him, with increasing passion, guiding his hands to her breast.*]

RODIN: Not here, my child . . . There's always the chance of visitors . . .

GWEN: Where then? Where? Please don't ask me to stop now . . .

[*She looks around rather desperately.*]

The wardrobe . . . why not? It'll be dark . . . private . . . no one will disturb us. We can close the door, leave the world outside. I was waiting for you. Now I'm ready . . .

[*She half pulls him after her.*]

[*They both exit.*]

[*After a while RODIN emerges. He straightens his clothing and hair which are rather dishevelled. He looks at the clay model, picks up the tool he was using and works on it a little. Then he turns as if to address GWEN.*]

RODIN: I must warn you . . . I am perfectly empty. Only my work fills me up. For years I have lived with the intrusion of those who want me. They force their way inside but find nothing. Then they complain about who I am and who I am not. You must understand this. I *am* my work. Everything is there. If you want a part of me, you must go to my work. Look — listen — touch. For there I am speaking clearly and giving what I have to give best. People come to me for a dream and what do they find? Just an ordinary man with an extraordinary sense of purpose. Years of single-minded concentration mean that I will not allow myself to be carried on waves of emotion or distracted by love or hate. To make sculpture, to draw, to let the human presence fill the senses — these are things I will not sacrifice. You may call me selfish, cold or arrogant — but I have paid my price — in grief, in bitterness, in tears, in envy and, believe it or not, in love.

To want too much is dangerous. It causes fatigue and sometimes madness. Where there is tenderness, you want it forever. I cannot permit myself to want anything that much — or anybody.

The only emotions I can allow myself are those which are of value for my work. Everything else must be sacrificed. Whatever you give me of yourself, I shall take only what is useful. The rest I shall throw away.

I am not prepared to justify my actions. Do not ever ask me to apologise.

If you are an artist, when you are *truly* an artist . . . *then* you will understand.

> [*He exits.*]

> [*After a while,* GWEN *enters, once more dressed as in the 'Self Portrait'. She goes to the easel, then to her paints. She picks up her palette, then puts it down again. She is clearly distracted. She walks to the table, sits down and begins to write. She speaks the words aloud as she writes. Here, as elsewhere, her French is often incorrect and spoken with a bad accent.*]

GWEN: "Mon cher Maître, Je suis si heureuse . . . si heureuse . . so very, very happy. Il faut que je vous dis c'est vous qui me fait heureuse. It is you who makes me happy. Oh my Master, you will be patient with me, won't you? Because, without you I won't be able to do anything which is good. Perhaps women can never do anything good except through the love of a man . . ."

> [*She gets up, goes to the mirror and looks at herself critically, as if for the first time. More sober suddenly, she goes back to the table, She looks at what she has written and almost angrily pushes it to one side. She then takes another, half-finished letter from the writing-case.*]

Ursula . . .

> [*She begins to write, speaking the words as she does so.*]

" . . . So much to do because, if I don't bring drawings to him, he says I sulk, so, what with drawing, posing, and translating, I feel as if I am getting quite thin. R. says I am too thin for his statue and that I don't eat enough, but I rarely have time to eat . . . Dear Ursula, is it last Saturday — I mean the sending-in day? I hope our pictures will hang together. I feel so lonely in the New English . . ."

[*She stops for a moment, looks into space, then continues.*]
"I have had some scenes with Rodin, and he is always adorable at the end. I see these scenes are necessary to him, but I wish they did not make me so ill."

[*She breaks off suddenly, stands, parts the curtain and looks out. Then she goes to the mirror and touches her hair. Suddenly dissatisfied with the effect, she smooths her hands over her breasts and turns sideways to look at herself.*]

*Work*, I must work.

[*She puts the writing-case back onto the small table. She goes to her palette and starts to prepare it systematically, almost ritualistically, as if the activity itself could help her to gain control. It is oil paint. The colours she uses are: Naples yellow, black, vermilion, crimson. She then selects about seven small brushes. Next, she goes to a small pile of prepared canvases, selects one (12½" x 10½") and carries it to the easel. She stands looking at the table and wicker chair. She goes to the parasol and adjusts it slightly. She straightens the cushion and rearranges the coat. She stands back to assess the arrangement, adjusts the position of the flowers, makes sure the curtain is hanging straight, then goes back to the easel. The objects thus arranged form the setting for: 'Corner of the Artist's Room in Paris (With Flowers)' (Taubman Plate 22). She begins to paint, at first with concentration, then stops.*]

Can a woman create works of art . . . a woman who loves . . who is in love? Or do both draw on the same store of energy, so that she can only do one or the other?

Oh my Master, when you are with me I feel so *alive* . . . as if I could move mountains . . . as if I could paint masterpieces . . . but then you are gone and I am only myself . . . [*Pause.*] I must not ask for too much. I must learn to be grateful and not disobey you. My heart longs to obey you. My senses cry out to obey you. You hold me in the palm of your hand. You are my Master, my beloved Master . . .

[*Light on* ROBERT *as* RODIN. *He reads aloud from* GWEN'*s letter.*]

RODIN:    "Cher Monsieur, Je ne sais pas quoi faire cet après-midi parce-que vous n'avez pas venu. I don't know what to do this afternoon because you haven't come. I'll put on the red dress if that's what you'd like . . ."

[*He take another letter from a pile.*]

"Mon Cher Maître, I wanted to say goodbye to you because I am sad this evening. Thank you for all money you have given me — it's much more than I can use — but I'll put it to one side. If you think of me sometimes, mon maître, think that you are my happiness and all that I ever wished for in life, because that is the truth. Goodbye, mon maître, your modèle, Marie."

[*He puts the letter down and picks up another. At first he seems somewhat bemused, then it becomes increasingly harder for him to conceal his irritation at the sheer number of letters.*]

[*reading*] "Mon Cher Maître, I didn't know what to do when I didn't find you today. Oh my dear maître, I didn't cry. I know that one must bear disappointment, that you want me to be brave. I wanted to cry, but I wasn't going to because you wouldn't want that. Oh mon maître, I love you, I love you. Oh what a joy it is to write to you. Now I am comforted that I'll see you tomorrow. I'm going to put the room in order. I'm going to eat well, as my maître told me to. I'm going to sleep as he would like. Pardon my weaknesses . . ."

[GWEN'*s voice, when she speaks, is strangely different: girlish, breathless, rapid.*]

GWEN:    St. Augustine . . . yes . . . yes, I remember. St. Augustine so much loved the . . . pleasures of the flesh, that it seemed to him that life without them would be unbearable. He only longed for that and, when he had to renounce it for God, he underwent a terrible struggle, which lasted a long time, and one day in a garden, he was desperate and he cried to God . . . [*usual voice*] Oh my God . . . my God . . . how long will this last?

[BARBARA *stands by the slide screen. Slide:* RODIN'*s 'The Kiss'.*]

TAPE:    ". . . but one of many in his complex life. The pain and ardour which Augustus had recognised in his sister . . ."

[BARBARA *wanders away, evidently disturbed. She stands*

*for a moment watching* ROBERT, *who is holding forth, then goes over to where* MOXI *is painting furiously.*]

BARBARA: *Was* she a great painter?

MOXI: She got through quite a bit of work.

BARBARA: That's not what I asked.

MOXI: How are you supposed to measure it? It's not about how much they're worth, buying and selling . . . It's the *pain* you see in them. The self-awareness. It makes them really powerful. But it's not the power of *force*. It's something more subtle. A sort of *quiet* power . . . Contained, disciplined, the result of real commitment and passionate care . . . not cold, but sharp, sharp as steel.

BARBARA: [*almost to herself*] If we're so strong, how is it that we so often appear weak?

> [*She wanders back to the slide screen, as if it might offer the answer.* GWEN *passes her and goes to the easel; she seems to stand looking at* MOXI's *work.*]

GWEN: [*voice on tape*] "Love is my illness and there is no cure until you come . . ."

TAPE: "Vulnerability, tension and unease are transferred to the subject of her portraits."

> [*Slide: 'Nude Girl' (Taubman Plate 30).*]

"The identity of the portrayer fuses with the portrayed. Sadness and longing are all pervasive . . ."

BARBARA: Work . . . I must do some work . . .

> [*Slide: 'Self Portrait, Nude, Sitting on a Bed' (Taubman Plate 26).*]

GWEN: [*voice on tape, reading from a letter*] "I am doing some drawings in the glass, myself and the room and I put white in the colour so it is like painting in oil and quicker. I have begun five . . ."

BARBARA: We mustn't stop working . . .

> [GWEN *sits on the couch and draws herself, looking in the glass as she speaks.*]

GWEN: Opened up . . . torn apart . . . like a book with its pages blowing in the wind. Oh Ursula, if you could see me now, you would hardly recognise me. If you could see me, you would take pity . . .

Love is a monster, devouring everything. It's a drug, an addiction for which there's no cure. I want him all the time, every moment of every day — and, yes, at night.

Especially at night. He washes over me like the sea; he fills every corner, every crevice of my body. There's no place he hasn't been, doesn't know, cannot penetrate. His tongue searches my mouth, his fingers reach up inside me. He has found me out. I no longer belong to myself.

[*Pause.*]

You know, I touch myself often. It seems to help with the pain. But just for a moment. Because the pain comes back — only sharper.

· [*Pause.*]

I should like to go and live somewhere where I met nobody I know, till I am so strong that people and things could not affect me.

Ursula — if you were here, what would you tell me to do? Be sensible? Be reasonable? Try to gain some sort of perspective? Can't you see . . . ? There *is* no sense. There *is* no reason. There *is* no perspective. Only this awful longing, tearing at me day and night . . . this madness. Nothing else. Nothing.

[*She stands for a moment. Then, as if gathering herself, she goes to the drawing, picks it up and looks at it. She speaks in a rather flat, automatic tone.*]

"The drawings . . . yes. I first draw in the thing, then trace it onto a clean piece of paper by holding it against the window. Then decide absolutely on the tones, then try to make them in colour and put them on flat. Then the thing is finished. I have finished one. It was rather bad because of the difficulty of getting the exact tones in colour and the hesitations and not knowing enough about water-colour. I want my drawings to be definite and clean like Japanese drawings. But they have not succeeded yet."

[*Long pause.*]

The cat ran away. Did I tell you? It was while I was lying in the bushes watching his house — *Rodin's* house. Did you know I did that sort of thing? You would be amazed. Alarmed. Shocked. The cat ran away and I spent whole days and nights looking for him. I lived in the bushes like a wild animal.

[*Pause.*]

Ida is dead. I wonder if you knew. Too many babies and

too much pain. It is hard to be the wife of a famous artist. My brother cried.

[*Pause.*]

"Oh my dear Master, I'm only happy when I'm asleep. I have gentle dreams and you are in them. Last night I dreamt that you came and we made love and the next morning I felt less sadness. I pray you to come. I've been ill for a long time — Prayer is my resource . . . the thought of God makes me happy . . ."

[*The following speech is spoken by both* GWEN *and* BARBARA. *It is not necessary for it to be synchronised.*]

GWEN: } Can't . . . can't go on. Feel so empty . . . lost . . .
BARBARA: } Nobody . . . nobody . . . Easier before . . . safer somehow . . . not expecting . . . not hoping. Torn open . . . torn apart . . . destroyed.

GWEN: I must try to be better . . . more patient. I *will* try. I promise to read St. Augustine. I shall remember my prayers . . . I'm sorry you did not like the red dress . . . I'm sorry . . . I . . .

[*She breaks down and cries helplessly.*]

MICHAEL: [*rushing up to* KAREN] You'd better look after your friend. For some unfathomable reason she's crying her bloody eyes out . . .

[BARBARA *too is crying.*]

[*Blackout.*]

# END OF ACT ONE

# ACT TWO

*The scene as at the end of Act One.*

*KAREN and BARBARA enter. BARBARA looks red-eyed and
exhausted. KAREN goes straight to the phone. BARBARA follows.*

KAREN: I'll get you a taxi.

BARBARA: I'll be all right now.

KAREN: Even so . . .

[*BARBARA touches her arm, pleading.*]

BARBARA: Please . . . I want to stay.

KAREN: Why?

BARBARA: Because my room's so cold.

[*KAREN looks mystified. A strange pause.*]

I . . . I don't know why I said that . . .

[*Light on MICHAEL as JOHN QUINN. He sits at the table,
writing. He has a New York accent, a very precise voice.*]

QUINN: ". . . to the bearer of this order, Miss Gwen John, residing
at 6, rue de L'Ouest, Paris, five hundred francs in bills,
as against the remittance of that amount by me to you
recently, and oblige yours very truly, John Quinn . . . "

[*He blots it carefully, then turns up another letter.*]

"July 29th 1910 . . . Gwen John, 6, rue de L'Ouest,
Paris, France: Dear Miss John, I was delighted when
your brother wrote to me that you had reserved one of
your paintings for me. I have just received a letter from
him in which he says that you put thirty pounds on it
and that he had remitted to you ten pounds at your
request. I am sending a Marseilles draft to him for ten
pounds to repay him what he has thus remitted to you
and I am sending you twenty pounds . . ."

[*Light on ROBERT as RODIN. He too reads from a letter.*]

RODIN: "March 27th 1914: Mon Maître, Today I can't bear it
alone . . . my heart and all my desires and feelings.
When I write to you . . . I am appeased because I no
longer feel alone . . ."

[*Light on QUINN again. His letter breaks into RODIN's
letter.*]

QUINN: ". . . one hundred pounds annually or in quarterly
payments of twenty-five pounds a quarter on the
understanding that you do for me one or two or three

paintings . . . This is not trying to monopolise your
work or anything of that sort . . ."

[*The letters criss-cross, merge. We hear first one, then the
other.*]

RODIN: "Mon Cher Maître, I have cried so much I can no
longer read. My eyes are painful. I am sad when I think
how you treat me, but happy when I think of my love.
You have no pity on my pain. But do as you wish. You
are my Master . . ."

QUINN: ". . . why the picture you ordered has not arrived . . . I
have been a long time trying to decide whether I should
send it and now I have decided not to send it . . . people
say it is so ugly, I am sure it is and I am doing one which
will be more agreeable . . ."

[GWEN *walks to the window. She parts the curtain, looks out
and sadly lets it fall. She looks unkempt, worn, distraught.*]

GWEN: I dreamt of him again last night. I was in a garden . . .
waiting for him in a garden. I stood beside a door. The
door opened and he came out. Of course he wasn't
alone. But when he saw me he came up and kissed me.
We sat down next to a pond under the trees. It was
evening.

[*She turns.*]

Yesterday I went for a walk in the woods. It was beautiful
. . . the leaves . . . the sunlight. Such a sense of calm. It
was as if I was surrounded by God, wrapped in his
kindness. Utterly at peace. Then, suddenly, I felt this
great rush of longing — spreading through me like a
fire. I could feel him, taste him, smell him — I was
engulfed, overwhelmed — there was no escape. Does it
lurk within all women, this monster of desire, lying
still, biding its time, waiting to rear up and destroy
everything? Or is it only me? Am I so utterly corrupt, so
totally lost? Or perhaps I *am* mad . . . just as my father
said . . . This thing inside me, growing like a cancer,
eating me alive . . . There was such pleasure in it . . .
Such ecstasy . . . my body transformed — water into
wine . . . touching the very highest place. No one told
me about the pain. I wanted you. I go on wanting you.
Waking and sleeping. No rest. No respite. Help me . . .
please . . . can nobody help me? Is there nothing . . .
nothing that can take away the pain?

*[Light on* PIP *as a young nun. She sings the Catholic Credo in Latin, very simple.]*

NUN: "Credo in unum Deum
Patrem Omnipotentem, factorem caeli et terrae
visibilium omnium et invisibilium.
Et in unum Dominum Jesum Christum
Filium Dei unigenitum,
et ex patre natum ante omnia saecula.
Deum de Deo, lumen de lumine,
Deum verum de Deo vero . . ."

*[At the same time* SISTER MARY URSULA *recites from memory.]*

SISTER: "When we make a mistake we must correct ourselves
gently and in tranquillity, without being angry with
ourselves or worrying ourselves. Let us fall on our
knees before God to say to him in a spirit of confidence
and humility, 'Lord have pity on me, for I am weak.'
Then let us rise in peace. Let us tie the thread of our
affections; let us continue our work . . . We must suffer
in our own imperfection to gain perfection. We must
have patience with our imperfections, working to
correct them. Those who can rule by their will over
their senses, over their imagination, over their desires,
their fears, are a race apart. How difficult but how
desirable to arrive at that state . . ."

*[*GWEN *walks downstage. She speaks in a low monotone.]*

GWEN: "Only at the point of despair, of resignation, when one
renounces the struggle, is one filled with joy and celestial
peace. We are in the midst of Him as fishes in the sea
. . . I will trust in God. I will ask God to make me fruitful
to the life I have chosen. I have chosen to be God's
spiritual child and he will guide me. I must work every
day. Each day is for work. Abandon yourself to God's
kindness . . ."

*[She stands perfectly still, then she too begins to sing the
Credo in a very quiet, almost childlike voice. As she sings,*
AUGUSTUS *walks up to her. She does not see him at first. He
stands and listens. Eventually* GWEN *sees him. She stops
singing.]*

Gussy . . . it's been ages!

*[They embrace. Then* GWEN *breaks away.]*

I've become a Catholic.

AUGUSTUS: You've done *what*?

GWEN:    I feel very sure about it. Please don't start attacking me.

AUGUSTUS:    Attack? What, *me*? [*Pause.*] No . . . that's good. Well, I suppose it is.
[*He wanders over to look at the painting on the easel.*]
Nuns, eh?

GWEN:    I've got to paint seven. It's a commission.
[*Pause.* AUGUSTUS *turns to her.*]

AUGUSTUS:    We want you to come home.

GWEN:    Home?

AUGUSTUS:    Me and Dodo. You're to come back to England. Stay with us at Alderney Manor. It's not safe for you here. Who knows what these German idiots will get up to next.
[GWEN *goes over to the painting, picks up her brush and starts to amend bits of it.* AUGUSTUS *watches, waiting.*]
Well?

GWEN:    You know me better than that.

AUGUSTUS:    I know you're as obstinate as a mule.

GWEN:    Remember the donkeys on the sands? Muffin . . . and what was his name — the dopey one?

AUGUSTUS:    Jock.

GWEN:    That's right. Jock. And the little fat one with the gammy leg. You always used to say he reminded you of the Mayor of Tenby.
[*They both laugh.*]

AUGUSTUS:    You won't come then?

GWEN:    It's good of you to ask.

AUGUSTUS:    Dodo will be disappointed.

GWEN:    Yes . . .
[AUGUSTUS *looks at her for a while.*]

AUGUSTUS:    Gwen, are you happy?

GWEN:    I have so much work to do.

AUGUSTUS:    That's not what I asked.

GWEN:    [*turning*] Are *you*?

AUGUSTUS:    Don't ever have time to think about it. Exhibitions, interviews, private views. Paint this, paint that, paint the other . . .

GWEN:    Well then, we're quite a pair . . .
[*They stand looking at each other.* GWEN *approaches him.*]
Take care, Gus. There are monsters everywhere.

AUGUSTUS:    *Monsters?*

GWEN:    You should seek protection.

AUGUSTUS: I don't know what the devil you mean, but I'll bear it in mind.

[BARBARA *comes up to the picture of 'Mère Poussepin' (in the exhibition).* ROBERT *moves over to stand beside her.*]

ROBERT: Bit of a fierce old biddy, isn't she?

BARBARA: She looks . . . *strong.*

ROBERT: She reminds me of you. Look at that mouth.

[*He touches the mouth on the painting, then* BARBARA'*s mouth.* BARBARA *knocks him away.*]

Hey . . . Hey!

[*He grabs her wrist.* BARBARA *turns away from him.*]

I'll come and see you tonight. After I've dropped her off. I'll tell her I'm having supper with my agent. You light a fire and I'll pick up some smoked salmon. You look as if you could do with a treat . . . [*Pause.*] Barbara . . . are you listening . . . ? Barbara . . .

[*This is broken into by* GWEN'*s voice. She is singing 'Ben Bolt', haltingly. At first we do not see her.*]

GWEN: "Oh! don't you remember the school, Ben Bolt,
And the Master, so kind and so true;
And the little nook,
By the clear running brook,
Where we gather'd the flow'rs as they grew."

ROBERT: You haven't heard a single word I've said . . .

[GWEN *appears. She is crying as she continues to sing.*]

GWEN: "On the Master's grave grows the grass, Ben Bolt,
And the running little brook is now dry . . ."

[*She breaks off.*]

First they took away the statues, one by one. Cold . . . strange how stone is always so cold. And you lying dead in the empty house. Silent. Still. Cold. Cold as marble. Cold as ice. My master. Why did you have to die? I wasn't ready. I didn't even say goodbye. At least while you still lived there was some hope, some possibility . . . but now . . . but now . . .

[*She drops to her knees.*]

I believe in God the Father . . . I needed you so much . . . never stopped wanting you . . . drowning in a great sea of longing . . . God the Father . . . God the Father . . . God the Father.

[*She starts to sing again, still on her knees.*]

"On the Master's grave grows the grass, Ben Bolt,
And the running little brook is now dry . . ."

[*She calls, in a child's voice.*]

Muffin . . . Muffin . . . trot along, Muffin . . . come on, Jock . . .

[*Light dapples the stage, rippling like water.* GWEN *jumps to her feet.*]

"We are in the midst of Him as fishes in the sea . . ."

[*She calls, in a child's voice.*]

Muffin . . . Muffin . . . Come along, Jock.

[*She looks around her, then moves forward. She speaks in a girlish voice, as if remembering.*]

"I bathe in a natural bath — the rocks are treacherous there and the sea unfathomable. My bath is so deep I cannot dive to the bottom. I can swim in it, but there is a delicious danger about it. Yesterday I sat on the edge of the rock and a great wave came and rolled me over and over . . . then it washed me out to sea and that was terrifying — but then I was washed up again . . ."

There are crabs and small shrimps in the rock pools. The sky reaches down to touch the sand. The sea goes on for ever . . .

"12th November 1918: Dear Mr. Quinn, I am going to live in a place in Brittany. It is such a wonderful place. If you could come and stay there for a time you would get strong. There is a wild lonely bay near the chateau . . . you can walk miles along it when the tide is low . . ."

"We are in the midst of Him as fishes in the sea . . ."

Muffin . . . Muffin . . . Gus . . . look at Jock! Look at him! As fishes in the sea . . . as fishes . . . as fishes . . .

[*She runs as if into the sea, lifting her skirt as she goes. The sound of the sea, growing louder, intensifying.*]

[*Brief blackout.*]

[BARBARA *wanders over to the tape.*]

GWEN: [*voice on tape*] ". . . one led perhaps in the shadow, but ordered, regular, harmonious . . ."

TAPE: "Her work gave her purpose. Religion replaced relationships. It is the dispersal of feeling . . ."

[BARBARA *walks away. She stands looking at* ROBERT. *She looks very thoughtful.*]

[*Slide: 'The Convalescent' (Taubman Plate 50).*]

[BARBARA *walks back to the tape. She listens intently.*]

[*Slide: 'Girl in the Blue Dress'.*]

". . . There is no underdrawing. She painted directly, applying the thick chalky paint in small patterned brushstrokes. The figure and its background are of the same overall texture . . ."

[BARBARA *walks quickly to* KAREN, *who is talking to* MICHAEL.]

BARBARA: I need to talk to you.

KAREN: Not now.

BARBARA: It's about the book. I've worked out what to do. [*very animated*] She'll go to the sea. It pulls her like a magnet . . . the waves, the sky, the curve of the shore. No boundaries. No limits. No straight lines or hard edges. She *must* go. To feel free. To feel safe again . . . Yes, of course . . . the sea . . . it's so simple . . . I . . .

[*She stops suddenly.*]

You're not listening to me, are you?

[*Pause.*]

KAREN: I don't know what you want.

[BARBARA *considers this.*]

BARBARA: Only love. Just a little unconditional love.

[*A long pause.*]

KAREN: There's never any half measures with you, Barbara. Whether it's work or relationships, everything has to be pursued to the bitter end. You're relentless. A sort of emotional steamroller. I'm sorry . . . but I just can't take any more of it.

[FRANK WEBSTER *comes up to the women as they stand confronting each other in painful silence.*]

FRANK: [*to* BARBARA] Someone told me you were a famous writer . . . and a card-carrying feminist to boot!

[BARBARA *never takes her eyes off* KAREN's *face.*]

BARBARA: Then someone was a liar. I'm not a famous writer. I'm still trying to find out whether I'm a writer at all. As for feminism, you'd better ask Karen. She's the expert . . . Excuse me.

[*She walks away.*]

FRANK: [*to* KAREN] Did I say something?

[KAREN *is still watching* BARBARA, *who goes urgently up to* MOXI.]

BARBARA: How do you ever know if it's really any good? Is it just a question of what 'they' say?

MOXI: You need to have your own criteria. It's nothing to do with other people. [*gestures around the room*] She was *never* satisfied. Whatever she did. She always felt as if she could do better. Even when people began to take notice of her work, she didn't want to show it. And she absolutely hated selling it.

BARBARA: Almost as if she'd done it all for herself . . .

MOXI: And why not?

BARBARA: Always to be measured by *them* . . . by their criteria. When all the time we know perfectly well what we are really capable of . . . It's a constant struggle not to lose confidence . . . it's a constant . . .

[*She turns as if interrupted.* GWEN *stands very close to her.*]
Struggle.

[GWEN *speaks almost as if to* BARBARA.]

GWEN: "Dear Ursula, I have been longing to hear from you lately. I think you might like to hear that I am all right . . . Like a plant that was dying and nearly dead and begins to grow again, how almost unbelievable and what joy it is to live . . ."

[GWEN *goes to the table and sits down to write.*]

[BARBARA *wanders aways from* MOXI *and stands looking at one of the paintings.*]

[GWEN *reads from the letter as she writes.*]

"Dear Mr. Quinn, I am quite in my work now and think of nothing else. I paint till it is dark and the days are longer now and lighter and then I read about an hour and think of my painting and then I go to bed. Every day is the same. I like this life very much . . ."

[*Light on* MICHAEL, *as* JOHN QUINN.]

QUINN: May I see the stuff you wrote about . . . the things you did in Brittany?

[GWEN *nods.* QUINN *goes to the drawings and looks through them.*]

This one's rather pretty . . . oh . . . and this one . . . No, take my word, they're good . . . very good. I've got a couple of shows coming up in New York. I want as much of your stuff as possible.

[QUINN *holds up some pictures, including a drawing of a boy.*]

I'll take these . . .

[GWEN *is surprised. She goes to see which pictures he has chosen. She picks up the drawing of the boy.*]

GWEN: I can't let you have this one.

QUINN: Can't? What do you mean . . . can't?

GWEN: I never intended to sell it . . . I . . .

QUINN: Sell? Who's talking about sell? We have our little arrangement, remember? I mean, what's the point of doing them if you never want to let them out of your sight?

[GWEN *looks for and finds another, similar, drawing.*]

GWEN: This one's much better . . .

QUINN: [*giving it a cursory glance*] Don't agree. Anyhow — this is the one I want.

[*He takes the original drawing.*]

That's settled then.

[GWEN *looks helpless.*]

Incidentally . . . I called in at the Convent. To arrange about the Poussepin picture. They're going to let me have it at last.

GWEN: But it isn't even finished. There's quite a few things I was hoping to . . .

QUINN: Seems the convent roof's been leaking for years. Anyhow, it looked finished to me. Trouble with you is you're never satisfied . . .

GWEN: But the nuns . . .

QUINN: The Sister Superior called it a miracle. God moves in a mysterious way, eh Miss John?

GWEN: So it would seem.

QUINN: I must say . . . I consider it your finest piece of work . . .

[*Light fades on* QUINN. GWEN *looks sadly through the remaining drawings as if something has been lost. Then she picks up the writing-case, goes to the table and sits down to write.*]

GWEN: "2nd June 1925: Dear Ursula, Tragedies have happened in my home lately and the cat I loved best has died *and* another. It has stopped me in my work and all the flowers I was going to do pictures of have passed now. There remain the acacia trees that I see from my window, but I cannot do them yet. If you bring home some work, we could have an exhibition this winter in London. I shall have enough I think . . ."

[*Pause.*]

"October 29th 1925: Dear Ursula, I find it difficult to think of an exhibition. These little drawings in colour won't do ... they're too small. I've got about five canvases that must be retouched. How many pictures go to the smallest exhibition and will the Leister Galleries take me for nothing?"

[*Pause.*]

"10th November 1925: Dear Ursula, Chenil writes that Gus would like a one-man show with me if it is agreeable to me in his Galleries in April. If *you* will exhibit with me I will write to say it is *not* agreeable ... "

[*During the last two letters* MICHAEL's *voice is heard on tape.*]

MICHAEL: [*voice on tape*] "New Chenil Galleries, Kings Road, Chelsea. Catalogue of paintings and drawings by Gwen John. Daily 10 till 6. May to July 1926.

Numbers 1 to 16: 'Group of Studies in Church'
Number 17: 'Road Scene'
Number 18: 'Portrait of a Girl'
Number 19: 'The Little Nun'
Number 20: 'Flowers'
Number 21: 'The Little Model'
Number 22: 'The Pilgrim'
Number 23: 'Girl Posing in a Hat with Tassels'
Number 24: 'The Letter'
Number 25: 'Mère Poussepin'
Number 26: 'Interior'
Number 27: 'Figures in an Interior'
Number 28: 'Study of a Cat'
Number 29: 'Enfants et Soeur'
Number 30: 'Study of a Cat'
Number 31: 'Little Girl'
Number 32: 'Study of a Cat'
Number 33: 'Enfant'
Number 34: 'Reading'
Number 35: 'Mrs Atkinson'
Number 36: 'The Road'
Number 37: 'Child with a Copy Book'
Number 38: 'The Blue Dress'
Number 39: 'Mère Poussepin'
Number 40: 'The Precious Book'
Number 44: 'Dorelia'"

[*During this,* GWEN *reads from another letter as she writes. This cuts across* MICHAEL*'s voice, which fades gradually to nothing.*]

GWEN: "15th July 1927: Dear Ursula, It's very lovely here. It's very quiet and peaceful . . ."

[*She gets up, moving with difficulty, as if physically weak. She takes a little Japanese doll out of a box on the small table, looks at it with pleasure, then places her hand on her stomach as though in considerable pain. She wanders to the window, looks out.*]

No view of the sea . . . we used to stand on tiptoe, Gus and I, but the houses were always in the way . . .

[*She potters weakly back to the doll on the table, re-arranges it slightly, then goes to the canvas on the easel. She begins to prepare her palette, using oils. She addresses the cat.*]

There was that little shop in the Boulevard Montparnasse . . . remember? The windows were always full of Japanese prints and dolls. I used to walk past there often. [*Pause.*] I know . . . that was years ago. Those lonely evenings. So much waiting, longing. [*stops for a moment*] It *is* possible to conquer desire. Of course, it takes a good deal of self-discipline — a determination to overcome all one's weaknesses. Work is a great source of stability. One should devote oneself to one's work. My Master always used to say . . . my Master . . .

[*She suddenly goes to the doll and picks it up.*]

But where are my manners . . . I should have introduced you to my friends . . .

[*She carries the Japanese doll to the wicker chair, where there are two rag dolls in print frocks. She holds them up as if to meet each other.*]

This is Dodo . . . and this is Dorothy. Dodo and Dorothy . . .

[*Looking at the dolls, she seems suddenly distressed.*]

Dorelia . . . why did I ever let you go? Those nights lying under the bushes, your lips stained with blackberries, your breath hot and smelling of bracken, your warm, fat little body. Dorelia in the black dress. I called you wanton, didn't I? Lost to me forever. My brother's wife . . . I said I loved you. Didn't you believe me? But then everyone loved you . . . Dorelia . . . Dodo . . . Dorothy . . .

[*She puts the rag dolls back on the chair and replaces the Japanese doll on the small table.*]

[*to the cat*] I'm going to buy you a present . . . a house with a garden. Perfect for cats! Well, it's not really a house . . . more a sort of wooden hut on stilts. It's just around the corner. Rue Babie. I expect you've been there on your travels. There's lime trees and acacias . . . lovely shady places to lie in the summer. We'll be quiet there — no one will bother us. No one will interfere. You see, selling pictures *does* have its uses. But no more exhibitions. And now John Quinn is dead, no one is waiting for my pictures. We will be all alone, you and I . . . alone . . . and left in peace.

[*She gets up painfully, goes back to the canvas and begins to paint.*]

[*Slide: 'The Japanese Doll' (Taubman Plate 61).*]

[*quoting*] "Those who can rule by their will over their senses, over their imagination, over their desires, their fears, are a race apart. How difficult but how desirable to arrive at that state!"

[*Pause.*]

A quiet round space inside my head. Everything in order. Everything under control . . . Nothing can touch me . . . nothing can harm me . . .

[ROBERT *goes to the hatstand and gets his cloak. He puts it on, also his hat, adjusting it in the mirror.* BARBARA *stands, watching him.*]

TAPE:      " . . . much needed money with which she purchased her dwelling in rue Babie . . ."

[*Slide: 'The House in rue Babie'.*]

"It was to be her retreat. It consisted of a mere shed, erected on half an acre of waste ground . . ."

WOMAN:   [*voice on tape*] "She had infinite tenderness, infinite sensibility, but no illusions . . ."

[ROBERT *turns and sees* BARBARA *watching him.*]

ROBERT:   Having dinner with my publisher. [*checks his watch*] Running a little late actually . . . I'll give you a ring . . .

[*A long pause.* BARBARA *looks at him steadily.*]

BARBARA:  Goodbye, Robert.

ROBERT:   I'll see you.

BARBARA:  No . . . you won't. Not this time.

[ROBERT *looks at her bemused and shakes his head in disbelief.*]

[*very quietly*] Everything in order. Everything under control. Nothing can touch me. Nothing can harm me.

ROBERT: Are you sure about this?

BARBARA: Yes, I'm quite sure.

[*She stands very still and does not look at him at all as he crosses to* PIP *and takes her by the arm. He looks across at* BARBARA *but she turns away, looking at the slide.* ROBERT *and* PIP *exit.*]

Nothing can harm me . . .

[*The sound of the Catholic Mass sung loudly and raggedly by a congregation in chuch.*]

[KAREN *as* VERA OUMANÇOFF *sits with her back to the audience. Next to her is* FRANK WEBSTER *as* JACQUES MARITAIN. GWEN *sits behind them. She is sketching* VERA.]

[*The Mass ends. Organ music.*]

[VERA *and* MARITAIN *get up, turn around and walk past* GWEN. GWEN *seems mesmerised. As they pass,* VERA *leans across to* GWEN.]

VERA: Do you often draw in Mass?

[GWEN *crumples the drawing and quickly drops it. She is confused, embarrassed.*]

GWEN: No . . . I . . . well . . . yes . . . No.

MARITAIN: I should not be surprised if it were considered a sin. What is your opinion, Vera? Do you think it is a sin?

[VERA *smiles.* GWEN *is completely captivated.*]

GWEN: Vera . . . Vera . . . Oh please . . . May I . . . ? Could I . . . ?

[VERA *and* MARITAIN *exit.* GWEN *leaps up, scattering her bag and its contents, pencils, etc. She scrambles to retrieve everything then hurries after them. The organ music intensifies.*]

[*Almost immediately, light on* GWEN *standing like a supplicant at* VERA's *door.* MARITAIN *opens it. He is not amused.* GWEN *looks like a naughty child.*]

I followed you home. I waited in the street trying to pluck up courage . . .

MARITAIN: We *were* aware of your presence.

GWEN: Rilke died today. He was a great poet. I knew him a little. He was a friend of someone I once . . . Endings and beginnings. God works in a mysterious way. May I come in?

[MARITAIN *lets her in, more courteously than warmly.* VERA
*sits at the round table, taking tea: very formal, very polite.*]

MARITAIN: The lady artist will join us for tea. In God's name, you
understand. I don't believe we have been introduced. I
am Jacques Maritain, a philosopher by profession and
inclination.

[*He offers his hand but* GWEN, *staring fixedly at* VERA, *fails
to respond.*]

And this ... [*gestures*] ... is my dear sister, Vera
Oumançoff. And you, madam, are ... ?

GWEN: I'm ... I'm ...

[*She suddenly sees a painting on the wall and makes a beeline
for it.*]

That's by Rouault, isn't it ... ? [*looks*] Yes ... I thought
so ... *and* that. Do you collect pictures, then?

MARITAIN: We believe that works of art executed in God's name
and not for the personal glory of the artist are worthy of
our respect, yes ...

GWEN: Oh ...

[GWEN *isn't sure what to make of this.* VERA, *sensing her
confusion, smiles at her.* GWEN *rushes over to her, ignoring*
MARITAIN.]

I've seen you in church every week. I followed you
home once before but I didn't dare to ...

[*She rummages in her bag.*]

I want you to have one of my drawings ... Here ...

[*She thrusts a drawing at* VERA, *who is completely thrown
off balance.*]

VERA: Oh no ... I mean, it would be quite out of the ...

GWEN: I shall be *desolate* if you refuse. It'll break my heart. Ever
since I first saw you I've thought of nothing else. I see
your face everywhere ... in the clouds, amongst the
leaves of the trees in my garden. I've been longing for
a chance to tell you I ...

[VERA *looks desperately at* MARITAIN. *He nods, then strides
up to take charge of the situation.*]

MARITAIN: Will you pray with us, Miss – er ...

GWEN: My name is John. Gwen John. But some people call me
Marie. [*to* VERA] I was a friend of the sculptor Rodin. *He*
used to call me Marie. And sometimes I called him
Julie. I wrote him letters "Dear Julie," as if he were my
sister. [*to* MARITAIN] Pray? But we've only just come
from church ...

MARITAIN: It is our custom to pray together every day, morning and evening. We ask God for forgiveness for all our frailties. We pray that our home may be a haven of peace, comfort and understanding . . . a place where art and philosophy meet for the greater glory of . . .

GWEN: [*to* VERA] Will you come to see my paintings . . . ? I live at 8, rue Babie . . . it's only five minutes walk. It's not very grand but . . .

MARITAIN: Of course, if you prefer to make your own devotions we will bid you farewell and . . .

GWEN: [*almost pulling* VERA] Will you come? Say yes. *Please.* I don't think I can bear it if I have to . . . When can you come? Tomorrow . . . ? Or later today? Please don't make me wait forever . . .

> [*Brief blackout.*]

> [*Light on* VERA. *She stands by the table on which there is a pile of freshly laundered pillow-slips.*]

VERA: Pillow-slips . . . On Monday they are laundered. Ironed on Tuesday. On Wednesday I make my inspection. Every Wednesday.

> [*She examines a pillow-slip.*]

Such a tiny hole, but in need of urgent repair.

> [*She puts the pillow-slip to one side and lifts out another.*]

My brother will not tolerate stains. A pillow-slip too flawed to be redeemed must be cast out.

> [*She pulls out a pillow-slip with a slight stain.*]

I am to cut them up to use as cleaning rags.

> [*She attacks the pillow-slips savagely with scissors. She puts the scissors down and touches her forehead.*]

My headaches start in the morning. Shortly after breakfast. My brother goes to his study and I to my medicine chest. [*laughs*] The doctor has ordered me to rest . . . but a house won't run itself.

> [*She laughs, then turns, and goes quickly to the window.*]

She is there again. In exactly the same place. Under the laburnum. She was there yesterday. And the day before that. Every day since we met. In the dark . . . in the rain . . . looking up at my window. [*Pause.*] Why are you watching me? What do you want? I have nothing to say to you. Nothing. And there is nothing I want to hear.

> [*She draws the curtains.*]

Direct sunlight. So bad for the mahogany.

[*She returns to the pillow-slips.*]

On Thursday I shall polish the glassware. The servants can't be trusted. My brother enjoys a glass of claret, a little port after dinner. [*Pause.*] In a *clean* glass. [*Pause.*] I, needless to say, am a total abstainer. [*touches her head*] Something pressing behind my eyes. Building up . . . clouds gathering before a storm. I wish I . . . I should never have . . . I . . . [*Pause.*] Christian charity . . . the simple hand of friendship. She looked so . . . so lonely. And that appalling coat! [*Pause.*] She was drawing me . . . all through the service. I could feel her eyes on the back of my head. Such strange eyes . . . sharp as pins. [*Pause.*] I saw the picture. I can't say I . . . it made me look so . . . so . . . Goodness . . . how the time flies! Sometimes I wish there were twice as many hours . . . sometimes . . . I could give her my old grey worsted . . . the collar is only slightly frayed . . . A woman cannot live alone. It has clearly made her mad. [*touches her face*] Portrait of Vera . . . no one has ever drawn me before.

[*The lights fade on her.*]

[*Light on* GWEN. *She stands awkwardly and speaks out flatly, almost angrily in a sort of self-parody.*]

GWEN: Chère Mademoiselle, I love you as I love the flowers. Chère Mademoiselle, I love you so much I dare not look into your eyes, but, like a small hurt animal, I need to be loved . . . chère Mademoiselle, chère Mademoiselle. Mon maître chéri . . . my love is my life. Are you surprised that I am not always reasonable and in control? Will you forgive me many of my weaknesses — will you? Dorelia, where are you? Chère Mademoiselle . . . I love you . . . I love you . . .

[*Light on* VERA. GWEN *stands, listening in shadow.*]

VERA: "Do you really have to write to me every day? I think not and even think it is injurious to your soul, for you are being too attached to a fellow creature whom you hardly know. You have strong feelings but they need to be turned towards our Lord and the Lady . . ."

[*Light on* GWEN.]

GWEN: "You told me my letter was too long. Too long for *what*? I think that souls in Purgatory must feel like me. I don't live calmly like you and the rest of the world. When you leave me, *you* will have a tomorrow and a day after and all the days of the week. For me it is the last day . . ."

[MARITAIN *stalks in. He goes up to* VERA. GWEN *stands by, like a dejected child.*]

MARITAIN: Every Monday. I have decided. Her visits must be restricted to one hour every Monday. This absurd passion must be contained for her own good.

[*He exits, giving* GWEN *a pitying glance as he goes.* VERA *turns to* GWEN.]

VERA: Jacques has decided that your visits must be confined to Mondays. You may visit me every Monday after Mass.

GWEN: [*catching hold of* VERA*'s arm*] But I can't wait seven whole days! It's more than I can bear.

VERA: [*removing* GWEN*'s hand*] It is God's will.

GWEN: Is it God's will that I should be so appallingly lonely? Is it God's will that I should never find anyone I am allowed to love? Is God really so cold, so cruel, so heartless? It says in the Bible — "God is Love" — so why must he keep us apart — why? Why?

[*She pulls at* VERA, *almost hysterical.* VERA *removes her physically.*]

VERA: You should not disturb yourself. You are not of a strong constitution.

GWEN: I *am* strong. I am as strong as an ox, as strong as a tree. Only life makes me weak — life and people. I have it in me to be the strongest person on earth — but people won't leave me alone — they're determined to destroy me.

VERA: God is wise, God is good . . . Perhaps you will take a little herb tea . . . Today we have camomile — so soothing for the nerves . . . and then I'm afraid I must ask you to . . .

GWEN: No — I won't take herb tea. I don't feel in need of medication. And as for my nerves . . . it will need more than camomile to soothe them . . . Here —

[*She opens her bag, pulls out a sheaf of drawings and thrusts them at* VERA, *then stalks out.*]

[*Light on* MARITAIN, *sitting at the table. He reads from his own book.*]

MARITAIN: "There are many joys not so paltry that we leave for Christ. We would love him very little did we not forgo for his sake things truly good and beautiful. And that is a kind of universal destruction, for it is almost as difficult, sometimes even more difficult, to detach ourselves from what we might have or might have had than from what we have . . ."

[*As he reads this, light on* GWEN *and* VERA, *standing. Their dialogue overrides his reading.*]

GWEN: What do you mean — never see you again —? How can you say this? What do you mean?

VERA: We need more time for our devotions . . . Jacques is so absorbed in his work. He has a new book to be published in . . .

GWEN: You can't do this. You can't! Every Monday, you said. Just for the hour. I didn't disobey you, did I? I never came on a Friday or a Tuesday. I kept to my side of the bargain. All those drawings . . . what have you done with them?

VERA: The drawings are perfectly safe.

GWEN: Where are they? Where have you put them?

VERA: I told you — they have not come to any harm.

[GWEN *grabs her roughly.*]

GWEN: Have you any idea? Have you any idea what this will mean to me? I told you — I can't turn my emotions on and off like an electric light.

VERA: [*gently removing her*] I will pray for you. You will not be alone.

GWEN: Pray . . . pray. What use is praying?

VERA: You mustn't fall into blasphemy, even in your grief. Remember — God is good.

GWEN: Is He? I begin to wonder. [*Pause.*] I brought you more drawings. If you still want them, that is. Or shall I take them away? You make me feel so . . . so foolish.

[*She puts the drawings down and stands facing* VERA, *desolate.*]

VERA: God be with you, Marie. The world is harsh. You must try to be strong. It's a lesson we all have to learn.

GWEN: It's a lesson I seem to have been learning most of my life. Goodbye, Vera.

[*She walks to the door, then turns.*]

Don't bother about the praying. I prefer to pray for myself.

[*The people at the exhibition begin to leave.* MOXI *is packing all her materials etc. back into the basket.*]

BARBARA: [*to* MOXI] Goodbye . . . and good luck. And please don't stop painting.

MOXI: I couldn't, even if I wanted to. [*Pause.*] What about you?

BARBARA: [*considers*] I'm . . . I'm feeling much better.

[MOXI *hugs* BARBARA.]

[SISTER MARY URSULA *goes up to* MICHAEL *and* KAREN, *who are standing by the table.*]

TAPE: "After Vera's death, the Monday drawings, as they were known, were found in a drawer, discarded . . ."

SISTER: Thank you. It has been most . . . inspiring.

KAREN: It was good of you to come.

SISTER: I feel very honoured to have been in her presence . . . She *was* here, you know. I felt it most distinctly.

[MICHAEL *smiles benevolently.*]

Thank you again.

[KAREN *extends her hand to shake hands.* SISTER MARY URSULA *takes* KAREN'*s hand and holds it, rubbing it slightly.*]

You're very cold.

[KAREN *is disturbed by this. She removes her hand.* FRANK WEBSTER *comes up.*]

FRANK: Must dash. Beryl's cooking my favourite. Chicken curry. Not too hot, but just hot enough.

[*He kisses* KAREN *on the cheek.*]

Take care . . .

[KAREN *is stroking her own hand, but watching* BARBARA, *who is escorting* MOXI *to the door; both are laughing.*]

[*to* SISTER MARY URSULA] Come on, Sister, I'll walk you to the Tube. There's a couple of things I've always wanted to know about Confession and Absolution . . . For example, if it's O.K. to do something bad, provided you then go and say "Mea culpa, mea culpa . . ."

[*They exit together while he rattles on.* KAREN, *still looking disturbed, runs back the tape.* BARBARA *picks up her coat and puts it on.*]

KAREN: I'll give you a ring . . .

[BARBARA *won't look at her.*]

BARBARA: There's no need.

KAREN: I'd like to.

BARBARA: I said "no".

[*A long pause.*]

KAREN: I don't know what the hell you want. Whatever I offer, it never seems to be enough. However much I give

you, you always ask for more. It's like walking in
quicksands. I feel as if I'm being sucked under . . .

BARBARA: I know. I'm sorry.

[*A brief pause.*]

KAREN: No, *I'm* sorry. I'm probably just tired . . . Look, please
phone me next week. Perhaps we could meet for a . . .

BARBARA: I'm afraid I'll be too busy.

KAREN: Doing what for God's sake?

BARBARA: Working.

[*Light on* GWEN. *She sits at the pine table. She is painting,
using gouache, on a very small piece of paper. It is more or
less a doodle, of palm fronds set against the background of a
draped curtain. Numerous other attempts at the same thing
litter the table and the floor.* GWEN *has difficulty in seeing
but works obsessively. After a while she gets up very slowly
and looks at what she has done. She picks up another version,
compares them, seems dissatisfied. She adds something to the
picture, looks at it again but is still dissatisfied. She sits
down and begins again. She is clearly frustrated by her
problems with seeing. She gets up slowly and gasps with
pain, holding her stomach.*]

GWEN: I should like to go and live somewhere where I meet
nobody I know till I am so strong that people and
things could not affect me beyond reason . . . People
are like shadows to me and I am like a shadow. I don't
think we change much but we disappear sometimes.

[*She walks slowly and with difficulty up to* KAREN, *who
now becomes* VERA. BARBARA *still stands close by.*]

VERA: [*to* GWEN] What did you want of me? What were you
asking for? Love, you said. What sort of love?

GWEN: Support. Warmth. Compassion. Something to take
away the pain. Someone to hold. Someone to talk to. At
night, or in the long, empty afternoons. Especially in
winter, when the light fails early. When the work
wouldn't flow, you could have brought me a cup of tea
as I sat drawing . . . you could have said, "Don't worry
. . . tomorrow it will all seem clearer." Afterwards we
could have sat together looking out at tulips you had
planted.

VERA: It sounds like a sort of marriage. What wives do for
husbands.

GWEN: And why not? All those men . . . cocooned in the loving
support of wives, lovers, sisters . . . and all those

women who might have done great work, if they had not spent their lives allowing *men* to be great. Where can *we* look if we are lonely . . . if we are to be supported, encouraged, understood . . . if not to another woman?

BARBARA: [*to* KAREN] I asked for something very simple and you weren't prepared to give it.

KAREN: You called it love. I thought of passion. I suppose I was afraid.

[MICHAEL *comes up.*]

MICHAEL: We'll leave the glasses till the morning, or we'll never get home . . . I'll just go and set the alarm . . .

[*He goes off.* BARBARA *and* KAREN *stand looking at each other.*]

KAREN: I suppose it's no good saying I'm sorry.

[BARBARA *stands, very still, very firm.* KAREN *looks at her but dares not approach her. After a while,* KAREN *exits.*]

[BARBARA *looks around.* GWEN *passes by her to return to the table and her drawing.* BARBARA *looks towards the table.*]

GWEN: "Not much to do with people. Perhaps nothing directly . . ."

[*She pulls the curtain aside and looks out of the window.*]
The acacia is beginning to turn . . . September.

[*She turns and speaks to the cat on the wicker chair.*]
There was some talk of war in the street today. Another war . . . I know, it's very depressing! How many wars can they fight before not one of us is left? Do cats declare wars or do you satisfy yourselves with terrorising small birds? [*fondles the cat*] What, talking of birds has given you an appetite? Then you shall eat! There shall be a dinner party for cats. I think there's still a little whiting left . . .

[*She kneels with great difficulty as if to put the food down, then gets up and fetches milk in a jug. She pours it out and sets it down, then slowly gets to her feet. She watches the cat with pleasure, then returns to the painting on the table. She sits down wearily and resumes work.*]
It is all to do with tone. The colours are the same but the tones are different. Infinite variations. Endless possibilities for change.

[*She gets up.*]
I must write to Ursula about colours . . .

[*She goes to the mirror and stands looking at herself. Then she turns suddenly, deciding.*]

I shall go to the sea . . . The wind blows fresher by the sea . . . Dieppe . . . yes . . . and afterwards, perhaps . . . [*to the cat*] Oh, don't worry . . . you'll have your food. Mrs. Bishop will see to that. Everyone eats far too much, the body doesn't need so much sustenance. But the spirit . . . now that is different . . . molten wax poured into an empty mould. My Master showed me how he cast his statues. Runners and risers. That's what they call the rivulets of bronze. Runners and risers. Dorelia was hot as fire. She would burn through you in a minute if you let her.

[*She wanders over to a painting and touches it.*]

So much left unfinished.

[*She goes to the table and looks at the array of little pictures. She spreads her hands out over them almost as if blessing them. Then she turns, goes to the hatstand, takes her small black hat and a black coat and puts them on. Picking up the milk jug, she bends with great difficulty to give the cat more milk. She gets slowly to her feet. She looks around the room, then, picking up her bag, exits, slowly, painfully.*]

[*The lights fade down.*]

[*A man's voice on the tape reads in French, but we hear the English translation concurrently.*]

TAPE:  "Le dix-huit Septembre, mille neuf cent trente neuf, deux heures trente minutes est décèdée, Avenue Pasteur, Mary Gwendolen John, artiste, peintre . . . celibitaire, domiciliée à Meudon, 8, rue Babie . . . "On the 18th September, Nineteen hundred and thirty nine, at 2.30 p.m. at Avenue Pasteur, deceased, Mary Gwendolen John, artist, painter, born in Haverfordwest, England [*sic*], daughter of Edwin William John, and Augusta Smith (both deceased), spinster, resident at Meudon, 8, rue Babie . . ."

[*Towards the end of this, light on* SISTER MARY URSULA *and* PIP, *as* FRENCH NUNS. *They are folding* GWEN'*s coat and other clothes.*]

SISTER:  Weighed less than a sparrow. Starved herself to death, if you ask me. Still . . . she didn't look like a beggar. [*looking at* GWEN'*s blouse*] Crêpe de Chine . . . this must have cost a penny or two . . .

NUN: They said she dropped down in a heap on platform one. Just got off the train from Paris. Didn't have any luggage or anything . . . Here, do you suppose she was anyone famous?

SISTER: Famous? No, I shouldn't think so . . .

[*The lights fade down slowly on them as* GWEN*'s voice comes up over this on the tape: it is strong, vibrant, full of energy.*]

GWEN: [*voice on tape*] Rouge phenicien is the colour of what we called wild geranium. The stems are dark crimson, the leaves are dipped in pale crimson just now. Earlier in the summer the leaves are vibrant green all over. Rose erythrine is a very beautiful and brilliant rose . . . Ochre jaune . . . yellow ochre . . . Cinabre clair, the green ball holding the snowdrop petals . . .

[*At the same time,* GWEN *walks forward. She speaks with considerable authority but quietly, evenly. She seems to speak directly to* BARBARA.]

If you want a part of me, you must go to my work. Look, listen, touch. For there I am speaking clearly and giving what I give best . . . You are free only when you have left all. Leave everybody and let them leave you. Then only will you be without fear.

BARBARA: But, the appalling loneliness . . . I'm so afraid . . .

GWEN: You must learn to be strong. Because no one will understand what devours you, this perverse and selfish passion, in the end more consuming than the love you have ever felt for any man, woman or even God. You will work till your eyes ache, you will work till your back breaks, you will work till your fingers bleed. You will forget to eat or sleep. You will call on no one and soon no one will come to call. You will grow silent, strange, intense, private. Every day your world will grow smaller but somehow clearer, brighter, more sharply defined, like a portrait painted on the head of a pin. Sometimes you will be drunk with it. Sometimes full of despair. You will always be utterly exhausted. Some people will undoubtedly call you mad.

BARBARA: So much pain . . . such a high price to pay. Didn't you ever ask yourself . . . ?

GWEN: I am not prepared to justify my actions.

[*A long pause. Then* BARBARA *makes a tentative move towards* GWEN. KAREN *stands in the doorway.*]

KAREN: Barbara ... are you sure we can't give you a lift anywhere?

[*Another pause.* BARBARA *does not take her eyes from* GWEN.]

Barbara?

[*Reluctantly,* BARBARA *turns to* KAREN. GWEN *stands now in shadow.*]

BARBARA: No. No thanks. I think I'd prefer to walk.

[KAREN *shrugs and disappears.* BARBARA's *eyes travel all around the gallery, searching. Eventually she goes to the 'Self Portrait'. She stands looking at it for a moment, then, reaching out, she very gently touches the face. She turns and again looks around. Then slowly, almost as if reluctant to go, she walks to the door. At the door she turns so that she is facing the audience.*]

[GWEN *crosses to stand beside the 'Self Portrait'. She stares straight at the audience.*]

GWEN: Do not ever ask me to apologise.

[*Slow fade to blackout.*]

# THE END

**Q** What do the following have in common:
Steven Berkoff · Michael Burrell ·
Anton Chekhov · Brian Clark ·
Barry Collins · Eduardo de Filippo ·
Keith Dewhurst · Nell Dunn ·
Charles Dyer · Rainer Werner Fassbinder ·
Donald Freed · Maxim Gorky ·
Richard Harris · Ronald Harwood ·
Franz Kafka · Roy Kift · Hanif Kureishi ·
Bob Larbey · Tony Marchant ·
Sean Mathias · Mark Medoff ·
Julian Mitchell · Mary O'Malley ·
Caryl Phillips · Manuel Puig ·
James Saunders · Anthony Shaffer ·
Martin Sherman · August Strindberg ·
Peter Terson · Heidi Thomas ·
Brian Thompson · John Wain ·
Hugh Whitemore · Snoo Wilson ·
David Wood · Sheila Yeger ?

**A** They're all playwrights, silly!

**Q** But what *sort* of playwrights?

**A** Amber Lane Playwrights, of course . . . .

Find out what you're missing out on by
writing or phoning for a copy of our free
catalogue.

**AMBER LANE PRESS**
Church Street, Charlbury, Oxford OX7 3PR.
(0608) 810024